CELEBRITY
STYLE SECRETS

Jacqui Ripley is a freelance journalist who writes for *Hello!*, *Now!*, *Cosmopolitan*, *Zest*, the *Standard* and *The Sunday Times*. She lives in East London.

CELEBRITY
STYLE SECRETS

An Insider's Guide to Looking A-List

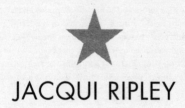

JACQUI RIPLEY

PIATKUS

The opinions and advice expressed in this book are intended as a guide only.
Neither the publisher nor the author is engaged in rendering professional advice
or services to the individual reader. If you have a medical condition or are
pregnant, the diet and exercises described in this book should not be followed
without first consulting your doctor. The publisher and author accept no
responsibility for any injury or loss sustained as a result of using this book.

Copyright © 2003 by Jacqui Ripley

First published in 2003 by
Judy Piatkus (Publishers) Limited
5 Windmill Street
London W1T 2JA

e-mail: info@piatkus.co.uk

The moral right of the author has been asserted

A catalogue record for this book is available from the British Library

ISBN 0 7499 2465 9

Text design by Goldust Design
Edited by Lizzie Hutchins

This book has been printed on paper manufactured with respect for the environ-
ment using wood from managed sustainable resources
Typeset by Palimpsest, Polmont, Stirlingshire
Printed and bound in Great Britain by Bookmarque Ltd, Croydon, Surrey

For John and Dylan

Contents

Acknowledgements

This book has not happened without the help of many people. I would like to thank all the experts who have contributed to these pages for their time and for imparting their knowledge, along with their publicity offices for their hard work behind the scenes in hooking me up with them.

Thank you to all my friends for their inspiration, encouragement and enthusiasm while I was writing this book, especially Jan, Jane, Wendy and Nadine. And my parents for their continual support.

Thanks to Alice Davis, my very calm and super-efficient editor at Piatkus, for immediately seeing the potential for this book and entrusting me to write 45,000 words instead of the usual 1,500 I'm used to writing for editorials.

Introduction

J ulia Roberts, Gwyneth Paltrow, Catherine Zeta Jones
. . . undoubtedly all bona fide A-listers and glamour
goddesses. But they didn't always look that way:
groomed, buffed and polished within an inch of their beautiful lives. Oh no, before those inspirational A-listers hit
stardom they looked, well, so normal. So what happened
between geek and chic? They hired experts, that's what.
Experts who gave them access to the hottest insider secrets
around. They purchased perfection along with their
diamonds.

The rise of celebritydom has been phenomenal: we want
to know what they eat, where they live, who they're dating,
where they shop and the name of the lipstick that they
wear. Heck, we even want to know where they have their
bikini line waxed! Nothing is sacred for too long when
we're talking celebrity. When people ask what I do, their
very next question tends to be 'Do you meet any celebrities?' There's even a newly identified psychological condition: Celebrity Worship Syndrome.

I don't profess to live my life like a celebrity. The only red
carpet I tread on is the one in my parents' hallway. But I am

privy to the tricks, slicks and picks that celebrities use to look lavish. It's that's six degrees of separation thing that comes into play. In my little black book I have the numbers of people who have preened and primed those famous women on the global celebrity stage. And along with some insider knowledge of my own, picked up from years of working closely with such people, I can give you the secrets of celebrity style.

Of course a celebrity lifestyle can be extreme, to say the least. So when reading this book, don't feel a failure if you can't keep up with some of their more demanding schedules, especially regarding diet and exercise. In a celebrity life there can be a fine line between enthusiasm and obsession. And sometimes once-grounded feet leave Earth for Planet Celebrity.

The true secret of looking good is becoming the mistress of your *own* celebrity, whether it's pulling out all the stops for a new look, opting for a happy medium, going the distance without going to extremes or making those small but powerful changes that can make all the difference in your life. The choice is yours.

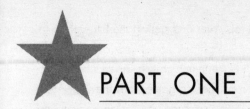

PART ONE

The scoop on fabulous-looking skin

'Here we glow, here we glow, here we glow' may as well be the chanting mantra adopted by many a superstar skin, as it looks as though celebrities employ a face fairy to fly down and wave a magic wand over their pores, blessing them with skin nirvana. Parties and premières, not to mention award ceremonies, amount to late night after late night and yet celebrities' skin never seems to suffer. Why?

Movie-star skin, like everything else in movie stars' lives, can be very high maintenance and that means a packed beauty itinerary of smoothing, brightening, toning, sloughing and buffing, not to mention the round of appointments with the skin specialist: the dermatologist. The most sought-after dermatologists are now just as famous as their clear-skinned clients, with many boasting their own skincare lines. These are the people who can make celebrities' skin look as though it's been poured from the fountain of youth. Although of course, in true celebrity style, when the pampered pore stars are quizzed on their complexion secrets they put their wonderful skin down to good genetics, drinking plenty of water and getting the full eight hours shuteye!

When it comes to fighting the march of time, A-listers believe it's never too early to play the anti-ageing game. They inevitably want their skin to be luminous, evenly coloured and lineless forever. And are prepared to pay for it – both in time and money. They know the value of a seriously healthy skin with a childlike glow.

Celebrities may well try to wrinkle their Botoxed brows (more of which later) over their complexions' fading glory, but they don't lose beauty sleep over it, as they know there are lots of things that can help bring back that fresh-faced appeal. Wendy Lewis is a top independent beauty consultant with offices in both London and New York. She is a true insider in the world of beauty. And as she explains, 'Achieving smooth and clear skin is within everyone's reach. You just have to know what to do and what to avoid.'

This is what this first section is all about: unpeeling bright ideas for skin to help kickstart fatigued pores and to bring even the most star-struck complexion a camera-worthy luminosity.

The basic steps to a movie-star complexion

Skin reveals the naked truth, so if you're feeling pooped before the party has even begun it will certainly show on your face. So how do you get your skin to beam and gleam and radiate brilliance?

Skincare, like a celebrity's personal life, can get kind of complicated, but contrary to popular belief, skin doesn't require an artillery of products – just a few tactical weapons, namely a cleanser and moisturiser, along with precise handling.

HOW TO DO FIRST-CLASS CLEANSING

Ask any skin expert to spill the secrets of fabulous-looking skin and they will undeniably hail cleansing as the ultimate prep step for putting that run-in-the-park glow back into your complexion.

'Superior cleansing is the single most important thing you can do for your skin and makes for a great base for your make-up routine.'

Sally Penford *at the International Dermal Institute that develops the Dermalogica skincare range used by Julianne Moore, Jennifer Aniston and Courteney Cox*

Sally Penford's message on skin cleansing is loud and clear: leave full-on stripping to exotic dancers! All you need is to keep your skin perfectly clean, without over-stripping it – then it will stay healthy and fresh-looking. In essence, cleansing is the most crucial step in skincare.

'The key to finding a skin-friendly cleanser,' Sally says, 'is looking for one that will match the pH balance of your skin – around 5.5.' But what exactly is pH? Well, think of it as part of the skin's inbuilt defence system, a system whose job is to protect skin from bacteria and help it retain the right amount of moisture. Depending on what you clean with, you can easily unbalance it. Tingling, redness and dryness are the superficial effects of a product that is more acidic or alkaline than the proper pH balance of the skin.

Sally explains that the worse thing you can cleanse your face with is soap. Soap is alkaline in its pH, skin is naturally on the acidic side, therefore soap will strip the skin of its natural oils.

'The effect of soap on the skin is like that after bathing. There is scum left around the edge of the bath that can only be removed with the use of a detergent. And it's the same for the face. Soap cannot efficiently be removed with water and if you use soap with hard water, it's hard to rinse off and will leave the skin looking dull.'

Sally Penford

Not the way to go for megastar skin!

Sally divulges the difference between flat and fabulous-looking skin is the number of times you cleanse a day. 'It should be four times,' she says. 'Twice in the morning and twice in the evening. Most people only do it twice a day, but the first cleanse will only remove superficial dirt. The second gives a deep-down "follicle" cleanse.'

Research from skincare experts Neutrogena reveals that when it comes to cleansing more than half of us hit the pillow with a face full of make-up, thanks to too many late nights. Dermatologists advocate that unless skin is scrupulously cleansed every night it will be more receptive to spots and blemishes caused by clogged pores.

The best way to cleanse?
Warm the cleanser in your palms, then massage it over your face and neck, leaving it to sink in for around 30 seconds.

⭐ **STAR BOX** *Breakouts on one side of the jawline could be caused by the telephone. Many people don't realise how often they're on the phone and how many bacteria are on the handset and how close it comes to the chin. Clean all the phones you use – including your cellular phone – on a regular basis with a disinfectant spray.*

For those who live in a hard water area, Penford even suggests this diva tip: use cotton wool pads soaked in bottled water to rid your face efficiently of cleanser.

A SKIN'S TRUE STAR: MOISTURE

Putting the moisture back into skin is just as important as cleansing for a blissed-out and glowy complexion. 'The minute you put on moisturiser, your skin looks good,' quips international make-up artist Daniel Sandler, who is often called upon to create make-up for the catwalk and has worked with many an actress. Whatever your skin type (more on this later), a moisturiser is essential.

'Pick a leaf and put it in water and it absorbs moisture very well. It feels nice and soft, it's thicker – it feels good. Get the picture? Out of all the treatments you can pick for your skin, hydrating is of the utmost importance.'

Dr Howard Murad, *Hollywood dermatologist to Calista Flockhart, Brooke Shields and Lucy Liu*

★ **STAR BOX** *It sounds a beauty cliché but drinking water really does make skin look and feel more supple. 'You know when you need to be hydrated,' says Dr Howard Murad, 'your lips feel dry and skin feels like sandpaper.'*

As any happy-looking skin knows, moisturisers not only make the skin feel nicer but also create a barrier that, when combined with the sebum on the skin, keeps moisture where it belongs and satisfies a thirsty skin. Moisturising to the max swells skin cells and helps fill out fine wrinkles. To get the maximum moisture drench into your skin, apply your lotion onto moist skin.

So now you know that efficient moisturising is the secret for naturally plumped-up-looking skin, how do you get through the moisturising maze? Simple: pick a moisturiser that marries your skin type perfectly, regardless of price or persuasive advertising.

So how do you know your skin type? Read on . . .

Skin types and conditions

Your individual skin type can be the cornerstone of good basic skincare. Misdiagnose your type and you could wind up treating it wrongly. But bear in mind, it's wise not to apply these groupings too rigidly, as skin requirements change frequently, affected by such diverse factors as ageing, climate, pregnancy or temporary skin problems. This is why celebrities pay someone to do the thinking on how their epidermis is acting!

Here the International Dermal Institute gives the lowdown on skin analysis.

Normal Skin
Appearance: Soft, moist and plump. Healthy glow and colour, fine texture, no open pores and little wrinkling

Cause: Genetic

Products: Gel wash-off cleanser, hydrating toner, lightweight moisturiser, hydroxy-acid exfoliant, hydrating masque, sun protection factor (SPF) 25

Oily Skin

Appearance: Shine, open pores, thick skin, little wrinkling. Possible blackheads and breakouts. If skin is combination rather than oily overall, there is an orange hue on the T panel (the 'T' shape running across the forehead and down the nose and middle of the face) only.

Cause: Genetic, hormone-dictated, incorrect product usage

Products: Antibacterial pH-balanced gel cleansers, hydrating toner, hydroxy-acid exfoliant, clay masque, antibacterial oil-free moisturiser, overnight medicated gel, SPF 15

Acne

Appearance: Oily with comedones (blackheads), papules (small bumps) and pustules, often red and sensitive

Cause: Genetic, hormones, stress, incorrect product usage, environmental pollution

Products: Antibacterial cleanser, hydroxy-acid exfoliant, antibacterial gel, clay, hydrating masques, overnight treatment, spot-treatment wipes, antibacterial oil-absorbing protectors, SPF 15

Dry Skin

Appearance: Visible dryness, tightness, tight pores, wrinkles, poor skin tone

Cause: Genetic, incorrect product usage

Products: Milky, creamy cleanser, hydrating toner, hydroxy-acid or abrasive firming serum or booster, nourishing oil-based moisturiser, eye cream, exfoliant, vitamin-rich creamy masque, SPF 15

Dehydrated Skin

Appearance: Flaky, tight on surface, very fine lines, oil and blackheads can be present
Cause: Lack of moisture, incorrect product usage, diet, environment, medication
Products: PH-balanced milky-based cleanser, hydrating toner, hydroxy-acid exfoliant, gel hydrating masque, silicone or lipid-based humectant protection barrier, SPF 15

Ageing Skin

Appearance: Wrinkles, loose skin, pigmentation, poor circulation, a combination of oily and dry
Cause: Genetics, sun, stress, free radicals, smoking and of course the natural ageing process!
Products: Milky, creamy cleanser, hydrating toner, hydroxy-acid mechanical exfoliant, firming booster serum, pigmentation treatment cream, nourishing moisturiser, eye cream, SPF 15

Sensitised Skin

Appearance: Can be hard to see; red, inflamed; irritated by heat, products and friction
Cause: Stress, friction, incorrect product usage, medication, sun

Products: Gentle calming cleanser, hydrating protecting toner, healing masques, soothing booster serum, protective barrier moisturiser, climate block

Pigmented Skin
Appearance: Brown or white markings
Cause: Sun, trauma, medication, stress, hormones, fragrances
Products: Milky cleanser, hydrating toner, hydroxy-acid exfoliant, hydroxy-acid booster serum, vitamin masque, pigmentation cream, moisturiser with SPF 25, eye cream with SPF 15

••

CELEBRITY PICKINGS *Hey, even the beautiful people suffer from spots. Cameron Diaz's skin has been so bad, she's even cancelled a première. Acne in adults is often stress-related, but using the right medication can help control breakouts. Look for the antibacterial ingredient benzoyl peroxide in skincare. If the condition is out of control, visit your doctor, who may prescribe antibiotics.*

••

Steps to a flawless-looking skin

There's good skin and there's perfect-looking skin: read 'flawless and poreless'. For flawless-looking skin, take these simple steps . . .

SCRUB A DUB DUB: EFFICIENT EXFOLIATION

'It's simple – radiant-looking skin comes down to efficient ammunition against dead skin cells. And that process is called exfoliation. It's celebrated as a quick fix to enliven a dull skin tone. When the top layers of the skin's cells are evenly aligned, skin reflects light for that all-elusive glow.'

Sally Penford, *International Dermal Institute*

When you are in your late teens and early twenties – and remember, many a successful star is way beyond that age – your skin is as good as it gets. It has adequate sebum to keep skin moist and there's plenty of collagen to plump it up. But the biggest asset has to be fast and effective cell turnover. It only takes up to 20 days for a cell to complete its cycle, meaning that the skin is in a constant state of regeneration and that the cells on its surface are fresher. As time ticks on, this process begins to slow. Dramatically. By the time you've eased into your forties, the process takes about twice as long.

So, to avoid thick and dull skin, exfoliate at least twice a week. Research also indicates that exfoliation can even increase collagen levels, helping to reduce the effects of ageing.

PREP STEPS FOR SKIN THAT'S ANYTHING BUT CAMERA SHY

Celebrities are no different from us when it comes to concerns about how to handle their skin. And they've discovered, via the best make-up artists on the beauty planet, that if you handle your skincare right, then your complexion won't need too much of a cover-up. You can use less make-up and your skin's natural beauty can show through.

CELEBRITY PICKINGS *Victoria Beckham is a classic case of this: in her* Spice World *days, her skin was subject to blemishes and breakouts and she gravitated towards a thick layer of make-up to disguise it. Today, after seeking professional advice and guidance, her skin can rely on a sheer coverage.*

The next step to super skin is getting to grips with the 'prep steps' which can get most complexions into pretty good shape. But it takes the right know-how to turn the good into the really wonderful. Here's how . . .

Foundation That Lights Up your Face

In the bad old beauty days, base came mostly in beige and far from being a one-slick wonder left skin looking caked and uneven. Today, foundations are super-smart and have fast-forwarded themselves into something resembling skin treatments. The best-looking bases boast almost miracle-like qualities to enhance your skin: light-reflective particles to give skin a soft-focus glow, sun protection factors to fend off damaging UV rays and antioxidants you would normally find sitting in a face cream.

But what's key when looking for the perfect-for-your-skin match? First, don't mistake foundation for a fake tan. A shade that's significantly darker than your skin tone won't make you look sun-kissed, just grubby!

'To mimic a (very nearly) naked complexion, work on a shade that literally disappears into your skin. If you're not too sure, go for one that's a shade lighter than your natural skin tone. And opt for the lightest texture your skin can get away with.'

Daniel Sandler, *international make-up artist*

For foolproof application, don't slap foundation on like paint – chuck out the sponge and finger blend into the skin. 'This warms up the foundation through body heat and therefore it spreads more naturally and smoothly,' says Sandler.

For the best coverage, start with less foundation than you actually need – it's easier to add more than to remove it – and work from the nose out towards the cheeks and hairline. Open your mouth as you apply foundation along and just below the jawline. You will automatically blur the give-away border between the face and neck. Never apply foundation down onto the neck – it looks dated. Brown ring marks on the collar are so not good!

Get the foundation right and you can skip the powder. It can easily give skin a parched and older look.

'Overall you want a moist look, not a wet skin,' says Sandler. 'It's important you control the foundation. Once you succeed, you'll be rewarded with a skin that looks as though it has drunk a pint of water: radiant.'

Five Savvy Foundation Buys: One is Right for You

Liquid: Ideal for oily, normal and dry skin. The most versatile, it's easily blendable and gives varying degrees of coverage.

Cream: Ideal for normal, dry and extra-dry skin. Often heavier in coverage, thanks to its intensive moisturising properties. Usually oil-based, so avoid this if you're prone to breakouts.

Compact: Ideal for oily and normal skin. Perfect for those whose life is busier than the casting couch. The powdery, matt finish delivers a light and sheer coverage.

Stick: Ideal for normal skin. Ideal for blemish-free skin. Just dab, blend and go.

Tinted moisturiser: Ideal for oily, normal and dry skin. Gives the lightest of coverage. Apply for a sheer and healthy glow.

Concealer: How to Do the Big Cover Up

What you learn fast as a star is that concealer is an absolutely must-have and nearly as basic as a toothbrush. Although it can accentuate the positive, it is just as important in camouflaging the negative. Concealer is designed to hide everything from morning-after-the-night-before eye circles to blotches, broken veins and pimples. But getting the shade, texture and application technique spot on (no pun intended) is crucial. A blob of weirdly coloured concealer can attract more attention than the flaw you're trying to cover up!

So what should be your prime pick? A light, blendable formula to bestow skin with a uniform tone is your aim. A common mistake when hunting out concealer is to pick one that's too light or too pink. Go for one that's just a touch lighter than your natural skin tone. Many make-up artists even use two concealers to perfect perfection, as the texture and colour of the skin under the eyes is different from that on the chin or forehead.

And when it comes to applying concealer, do like the professionals do: apply it to either side of the nose, under the eyes, especially towards the corners if bluish veins are visible, and to any broken veins. Pat it on gently, rather than rubbing it in. Blend out the edges with a Q-tip.

To send under-eye circles into professional hiding use a concealer mixed with a dab of eye cream. Uncustomised concealer under the eyes can make them look crêpey and more tired. Apply a very thin coat to the darkest part of the circle and pat with your finger to blend.

The Ultimate Camouflage List

To mask almost any imperfection efficiently it's critical to know what to buy. Like foundation, there are many varieties of concealer from which to choose:

The pot: The mother of all concealers, as it's the thickest, which makes it the ultimate make-up tool for covering arrogant spots, dark shadows and uneven pigmentation. For a more natural look, you can always mix in a little moisturiser.

The wand: This liquid concealer comes with a sponge-tip or brush applicator so you don't have to stick your finger into the make-up. Although not truly effective at masking dark circles, as the formula can be a bit on the sheer side, it's superb for use in hard-to-reach crevices like the side of the nose.

The tube: Creamier than liquid, a squeeze-out concealer offers good light coverage. Ideal for chucking into your purse.

The stick: Shaped like a lipstick bullet, it makes dotting on coverage easy. The same can be said for a concealer pencil.

Cheek-to-Cheek Colour: How to Blush Up

Make-up artists to the stars know that giving cheekbones some well-deserved attention can supercharge your glow and bring your face back to life like nothing else. To achieve that flushed-beneath-the-skin-surface smoulder you need to flush up with the right colour and formulation. That's one that looks as natural as possible. The mission is to try and recreate the slight flush that excitement brings – like winning an Academy Award!

Blush can also be a secret weapon for distracting attention from under-eye circles. Simply bring your blush closer up to your eye, to where the circles end and cheeks begin. The problem will be instantly less noticeable.

When it comes to applying blush to the cheeks, you can forget about old techniques of contouring or sweeping colour all the way to the temples. Modern blush is applied carefully to the apples of the cheeks.

'Apply blush directly onto the skin with your fingers. Place it where you would blush naturally: right in the middle of the cheek. Always blend from the centre to the ear, otherwise you push the skin in an unnatural way.'

Laura Mercier, *make-up artist to Gwyneth Paltrow, Susan Sarandon and Madonna*

Bronzer can also be used in the same way as blush. It gives the complexion a warm glow and is a great temporary stand-in for self-tanner.

Choosing Your Colour

If your skin is fair: Go for pale pink or peach.

If your skin is medium: Try warm pinks or pinks with a subtle touch of red.

If your skin is dark: You need deep colours that are bright enough to liven up the face. Look to plum, rust or red.

Shopping for perfect skin

I s the answer to perfect skin at a counter near you? Or is there someone who can help you find it?

Celebrity or not, we are all born with perfect skin. And that's skin that works. To help hang onto that pore perfection, or to get it back, celebrities spend a lot of their free time hanging out at their Hollywood skin doctors in the hope of finding new elixirs to arrest the much-dreaded ageing process.

Los Angeles dermatologist Dr Howard Murad has top billing with many celebrities and frankly says don't believe all you see, as the camera can lie when it comes to a celebrity's complexion. He reveals, 'The truth is when you see these gorgeous famous women on the cover of magazines they are airbrushed to poreless flawlessness and when on the screen they are bathed in the best technical light to flatter. Collectively, this can make an ordinary skin feel inadequate. But ignoring this, celebrities spend more time than most attending to their skin, as it's always up for public and critical inspection.'

Murad's philosophy is 'internal skincare', by which he means nutritional supplements in addition to the application of topical products.

> 'If you apply vitamin C directly on the skin, it affects the outer layer. Taken internally, it affects the inner layer. It's ideal to do both.'
>
> **Dr Howard Murad**

Every skin doctor's advice is wide-ranging, especially in Hollywood, where many of these white-coated skin boffins are now famous in their own right. These guys with their impeccable pedigrees (both in qualifications and name-drop list) can boast their own face creams bursting with a whole cocktail of vitamins, minerals and face-saving technology.

And it's technology that's changing incredibly fast. Comparing a pot of cold cream to today's turbo-charged anti-ageing moisturiser is like pitching a Filofax against a do-it-all PalmPilot. So you should aim to update your skincare knowledge as regularly as leading men swap their leading ladies.

So, with dermatologists' offerings, plus what's available on the chemists' shelves, what's a 'real face' to choose? Here's the low-down on the star ingredients to look for in your moisture pots.

The SOS (Save our Skins) Hit List

Alpha Hydroxy Acids: AHAs, found in sugar, milk and fruit, have been the most important scientifically proven skin smoothers in decades.

Alpha Lipoic Acid: A key antioxidant used in dermatologist Nicholas Perricone's Cosmeceuticals skincare range. Skin doctor to Julia Roberts, Perricone describes this ingredient as a 'universal antioxidant', hailing it as 400 times stronger than vitamin E and C combined. 'Ageing is optional,' he says.

Copper: The third most common trace element in the body and a known collagen stimulator, copper provides a rigorous defence against environmental and lifestyle free-radical damage. It helps the body 'remember' its youthful appearance by actively promoting collagen and elastin renewal.

Green Tea: Provides antioxidant and anti-irritant benefits, helping to diminish lines. The polyphenols from green tea are said to protect skin from UVB damage.

Liquorice Extract: Helps to brighten and even out skin tone to deliver skin with an awakened vibrancy.

Phytoestrogens: Otherwise known as isoflavones, these impersonate the effects of the female hormone oestrogen, which declines in peri-menopausal and menopausal skin, leaving it dry and less elastic. Taking natural 'hormones' including soy and wild yam keeps your skin hydrated and toned.

Pomegranate Extract: 'A proven SPF booster and antioxidant to age-proof the skin,' quips Dr Howard Murad.

Sucrose: Yep, it's the stuff we shouldn't touch for our hips, but has been found to be good for our pores. A natural sugar antioxidant, it helps to relieve uncomfortable skin conditions such as itchiness or tightness. Makes a great double act when combined with green tea to help counteract long-term visible signs of ageing.

Vitamin A: Retinol is the chemical name for vitamin A. It helps thin out the thicker layer of dead cells by increasing the rate of cell turnover, exfoliating, stimulating growth of new blood vessels and promoting production of collagen and elastin.

Vitamins C and E: Preventative as well as restorative, this powerful antioxidant duo works synergistically and helps retard the formation of free radicals, the molecules that cause the breakdown of the collagen and elastin of skin and therefore the formation of slack skin and wrinkles.

White Tea: Rich in polyphenols, it helps neutralise free radicals and has been proven to be more effective at neutralizing free radicals than green tea.

 STAR BOX *When shopping for skincare, take note of the label. The active ingredients will always be at the top.*

SKIN CLONING

Isolagen sounds like something from a science-fiction movie, but it is a remarkable treatment that cultures your own skin cells so that they can be used to reduce the visible ageing process – if not now, then in the future. First off, a small skin sample is taken from behind the ear. Then, in the laboratory, fibroplasts (collagen-producing cells) are replicated. It takes about eight weeks for a sufficient quantity to be grown. When injected into the skin, the cells stimulate the body's natural collagen production. Over the next few weeks the skin appears more youthful, though it takes 18 to 24 months for the full effect to be apparent. Tests in the US have shown that women have kept their younger-looking face for some five years after treatment. If further improvements are required in the future, never fear. Your collagen-producing cells have been cryogenically preserved, frozen at the same age as when they were collected. Injecting youth has now become a reality!

★ **STAR BOX** *The one area of your face that doesn't wear well is around the eyes. The skin here is a quarter of the thickness of skin on the rest of the face and consequently more delicate. Protect with the stars' favourite: wraparound dark shades and a good eye cream with active ingredients.*

Putting off your first facelift

When it comes to fighting the march of time, faces that are up close and personal with the flashgun are as prepared as any army. They believe preventative skincare tactics are vital in the war against the wrinkles.

Every woman from her thirties onwards would generally like to look 10 years younger than detailed on her passport. And believe me, some celebrities seem to stick at 37 years old for 10 years! But in the image-driven society we live in today, is it any wonder that wrinkles are literally frowned upon?

The prime-time beauty peak for skin is between the ages of 20 and 30. What happens after this?

The deepest and thickest layer of skin is called the dermis and this provides the strength and structure of the skin. As age creeps up, the dermis naturally becomes thinner and weaker, causing skin to sag. Exposure to UV light speeds this process up, causing skin to lose its resilience and become wrinkled. The production of collagen and elastin

– the skin's inner mattress – starts to slow down too. Skin is less well anchored, facial features start to appear fuller and contours lose definition. As the structure of the collagen bundles becomes uneven, the skin's foundation begins to crumble.

This may not be the happy ending a leading lady desires for her skin, but although you can't turn the clock back, you can try your darndest to give your skin the protection it deserves. One way is to avoid the 'face wreckers'.

LIFE'S FACE WRECKERS

Celebrities tend to work hard but play hard, and lifestyle plays an enormous and often underestimated part in extrinsic ageing.

Smoking

Smoking just half a packet of cigarettes a day for two years can double your number of premature wrinkles, according to American research. Smoking not only encourages expression lines around the mouth and eyes but also activates free radicals, destroys vitamin C and starves the cells of oxygen. The result is skin that is sallow and leathery looking. Research carried out by American dermatologist Dr Karen Burke revealed smokers aged 40 could have the same number of wrinkles as a 60-year-old.

Sun Worshipping

It's well documented that sunlight is responsible for 80 per cent of premature ageing. In no uncertain terms it produces fine lines, brown spots, deeper wrinkles and leathery skin texture. Wearing a sun protection factor every single day – dermatologists advocate dipping no lower than an SPF15 – is the single most meaningful thing you can do now to save the cost of a facelift later.

> ★ **STAR BOX** *Check with your doctor that any oral medication you may be taking doesn't cause sun sensitivity. Birth-control pills, tetracycline and Retin-A, for example, will make your skin more vulnerable to sunburn.*

Drinking

And I don't mean herbal tea! Drink in moderation is fine – a celebrity is never the toast of the town without a glass of bubbly – but too much alcohol dehydrates the body, robbing cells of moisture and causing premature ageing. Drinking also depletes the body of nutrients, in particular vitamins A, B, C, magnesium, zinc and the essential fatty acids.

Exercise Shy

Let's face it, most celebrities aren't exercise shy, as they know exercise is the route to an A-list body. But for those of us who don't have three hours a day to make best friends with the treadmill, a brisk walk can be enough to improve circulation to the skin, feeding cells and making the complexion look radiant.

Worry

Every time you frown, you risk making the furrows

between your brows a permanent fixture. Any repeated facial movement can leave grooves in the skin. Perhaps that's why so many stars chill out with yoga. The Lion Pose, for instance, can help facial muscles become stronger and more defined over time. Sit on your heels, lean slightly forward and exhale forcefully through your mouth, making an 'aaah' sound. At the same time, stretch your tongue out and down and raise your eyes up towards the brows. Hold the pose for as long as you can.

HOW NOT TO LOSE FACE

In life – even lives seemingly sprinkled with gold dust – you can rarely have your cake and eat it too. And that's so true when it boils down to body politics. Unfair as it seems, there comes an age when you have to pick between keeping a complexion like a juicy ready-to-pick peach or a toned and high butt. There have been many celebrities who have been willing to sacrifice their full faces for super-svelte bodies, while others have kept their cherubic faces along with their womanly curves. Catherine Deneuve once said she sacrificed her figure in order to save her face. It's paid off: she's one of the faces of L'Oréal.

Getting skinny can take its toll on your face – dropping more than a stone, for example, can make you go jowly. But by far the worst ageing culprits are fad dieting, whether fat-free, carb-free or liquid filled, and yo-yo dieting. These can make your face look gaunt and lacklustre faster than smoking, sun exposure and stress. The endless cycle of gaining and losing weight stretches the skin to the point of no return and elasticity drops significantly. At some stage, it just won't bounce back anymore.

'A young person can cope with facial fat loss because their skin is elastic and will adjust itself to the volume reduction. However, past middle age this is no longer possible and skin will become loose, particularly in the mid-face, jowls and neck. Hence the scraggy look many body-obsessed celebrities can wind up with.'

Jan Stanek, *leading cosmetic surgeon*

And extreme dieting isn't the only face wrecker you have to worry about. Serious jogging can also have a detrimental effect on the face simply because it makes you very lean, with an overall loss of subcutaneous fat (fat that's deep under the skin, giving it that even contour of youth) and therefore support to facial skin.

The solution? Find the 'Botox' of exercise – that's a regime that takes the strain away from the facial muscles in order to curb frowning but still works hard enough to firm up your assets. For cardiovascular exercise stick to swimming, cycling and power walking. And for those who crave the treadmill, don't over-run, simply walk fast up an incline to really work your rear view.

CELEBRITY PICKINGS *Celebrities spend precious time seeking out age-prevention facials. Two of the most popular treatments are vitamin C facials and collagen masks. Both procedures have been described as 'the push-up bra for the complexion'. Madonna and Renée*

Zellweger are also fans of rescuplting facials (a machine is used that sends electrical currents to retrain the muscles to prevent sagging).

THE WRINKLE PICKERS: FOR WHEN THE CREAMS DON'T WORK

A celebrity ultimately wants rested-looking skin. That's a skin that mimics all the benefits of a good night's sleep. Glowing and blemish-free. But it's a sad fact of life that once past the age of 35, a complexion that was once so radiant will begin to look tired and tested. Time and emotion (and there's plenty of that with Oscar speeches) create lines on celebrities' faces they'd rather not pay tribute to. And few of them can merrily laugh off wrinkles, uneven pigmentation and a dull texture without wanting to do something about it. There comes a point when they start to feel dissatisfied with the signs of the advancing years and realise that all the anti-wrinkle creams in the world won't give them back smoother features.

'With this in mind, growing medical knowledge and advances in dermatology have brought sophisticated non-surgical treatments such as injectables, laser and chemical peels into being,' states British-born cosmetic surgeon Laurence Kirwan, who divides his time between London and Connecticut and whose mouth is firmly zipped when it comes to stars he treats!

These treatments claim not to alter features as such but improve on them to give a fresher-looking complexion.

'A whole menu of procedures can now literally whip years off your face and give you fabulous skin at every age. The signs of ageing can now be reduced or eliminated with little if any discomfort, and for the most part there's little or no "downtime" from work and social life.'

Laurence Kirwan, *cosmetic surgeon*

Celebrities see these non-invasive procedures that bridge the gap between skincare therapists and cosmetic surgery as well-invested maintenance rather than an act of vanity – although it has to be said that some stars have gone over the top and wound up with a mask-like complexion. Certain film directors now refuse to cast actresses with Botox, deeming them frozen. Contrary to this, a personal ongoing relationship with a cosmetic 'derm' does seem to be the stars' latest gotta-have. So what are the latest cosmetic procedures?

COSMETIC PROCEDURES THAT DELIVER THE YOUTH FACTOR
Botox
This readily-available wrinkle eradicator (full name botulinum toxin) has become known as 'the friendly poison'. Injecting a tiny amount directly into the muscles below expression lines temporarily paralyses them, putting wrinkles into submission for four to six months. Botox can treat furrowed brows, crow's feet, lines in the neck, vertical marionette lines that run from the outside corner of the mouth to the chin and lines on the chest. It's also used for excessive sweating and can be injected under the arms, into

the soles of the feet – guaranteeing starlets don't slide out of their sling-backs – and into the palms of the hands. It can also be used to stop anti-social blushing. Injecting small dots of Botox under the skin of the cheeks stops the nerve connection between the sympathetic nerve system and the blood vessels.

Facial Fillers

The biggest part of a star's body is sometimes their lips and that can be attributed to fillers. Collagen, Hylaform, Restylane and Perlane are all branded temporary skin fillers that can either pump up a pout or soften wrinkles in the forehead and around the eyes and mouth. Their aim is to help replace skin's natural suppleness. They can also be used on the deep lines that develop between the nose and corners of the mouth. Temporary skin fillers last between three to six months. If a good result is obtained with a temporary procedure, the use of permanent filler such as Artecoll could be considered.

Skin Peels

These are big news in the quest for a brighter-looking complexion. Sounding like something Dr Crippen would specialise in, peels literally remove surface skin. They come in different strengths. Superficial peels such as glycolic acid, otherwise known as fruity peels, are derived from natural fruit and sugar cane and work well primarily on very fine lines and rougher scaly blemishes. Medium peels that use trichlorocetic acid (TCA), which is more powerful than glycolic acid, are generally more effective on damage that nestles in the deeper layers of the skin. And then there are deep peels that use phenol. These are aggressive and 'downtime' can be up to three months. The payoff? The results can be dramatic and long-lasting.

··

CELEBRITY PICKINGS *It's been revealed that old-time Hollywood movie stars such as Bette Davis and Marilyn Monroe used to secretly tiptoe to quiet places outside Tinseltown to undergo face peeling. These 'peelers' were eventually named and shamed and put an end to by a politically correct medical establishment. One of the last remaining peelers traded her formulation to a well-known plastic surgeon in return for a facelift. He later published the secrets of the peel in the plastic surgery journals. Known as the Baker Peel, today it has become a widely used modified TCA peel otherwise referred to as Easy Peels.*

··

Microdermabrasion

Also known as 'mechanical exfoliation' or 'a speed peel', this non-surgical, non-chemical and non-invasive procedure is sought by many celebrities, including Madonna and Cameron Diaz, for a fast and painless fresher-looking complexion. The skin is blasted using diamond-hard ultra-fine aluminium oxide crystals. The crystals are then vacuumed back up along with the exfoliated layer of skin, plumping up collagen along the way. The result? An immediate glow to go.

Fat Transfer

Instead of injecting collagen to help smooth out nose-to-mouth lines, hollow cheeks or thin lips, you can use your own (surplus) fat from your stomach, buttocks, hips and outer thighs – proving that if you've got too much fat in your bum cheeks you can always move it up to the apples of your cheeks! This procedure can be one of the best remedies to smooth away any gauntness and is a proven treatment to pep up worn-looking skin. An extra advantage is that there's no risk of an allergic reaction or rejection, as the fat comes from your own body.

Laser Resurfacing

Doctors have literally been dazzled by the power of their lasers in the fight against wrinkles. Laser treatment resurfaces the skin, literally vaporising thin layers of skin tissue to erase wrinkles, fine lines, age spots, lipstick lines and sun damage. There are five basic laser treatments but the two most frequently used are the CO_2 laser and Erbium: YAG laser. The laser light is 'painted' evenly over the skin and stimulates the replacement of older damaged skin with younger and smoother skin. The lasers are so accurate in their pinpointing that deeper wrinkles and scars can be selected and treated separately.

CELEBRITY PICKINGS *If you thought bright-eyed stars just relied on eye creams, think again. They commonly tip the wink to a blepharoplasty operation, otherwise referred to as 'an eye job'. One of the most popular cosmetic procedures around, this involves having excess fat* *skilfully cut away from above and below the eyelids to lose puffiness and eyebags and raise the brows.*

20 SECRET SKIN TIPS

1. In winter we spend more time in centrally heated rooms and eat less fresh food. It's little wonder our skin can feel dry and neglected. Combat this by rethinking your moisturiser. A change of texture may be just what your skin needs to feel comforted.

2. Alternatively, try this nurturing DIY facial treat for dry skin. Mix an egg yolk with a quarter of a teaspoon of honey and three dessertspoons of goat's yoghurt. Apply to the face and leave for 15 minutes. Rinse off thoroughly.

3. If you have oily skin, look for natural ingredients such as ylang ylang, mint and camphor. They help sedate active sebaceous glands.

4. Never, never pick spots. Constant picking disrupts the pH balance of the skin and breaks down its natural protection.

5. Carry blotting powders around in your bag. Early afternoon is when sebum levels in your skin peak and you wind up looking shiny.

6. If you're confused about your skin type, booking in for a professional facial can be a worthwhile investment. You'll be told all you need to know and you can get to grips with your complexion immediately.

7. To boost healthy skin cell growth, take a six-week course of cod liver oil every season.

8. Invest in a primer. As well as acting as a make-up base, primers give the skin a subtle luminescent quality.

9. Do not use flannels to remove cleansers. Unless you use a clean one every time they can harbour bacteria.

10. There's a clear connection between stress and skin problems. Stress may invite dry skin conditions such as eczema. If you're concerned, visit your doctor for advice.

11. Always wash your hands before cleansing. Practical advice, but it's surprising how many people don't!

12. Night creams can really give troubled skin extra beauty points. Research shows that skin is more receptive and cell renewal is highest when resting and free from the onslaught of pollutants.

13. Always cleanse your face before applying a face mask. Applying a mask on top of a dirty face will stop its beneficial properties from being absorbed.

14. Good skincare never stops at the jaw. Whatever you do for your face, do for your neck too.

15. If you are using an eye cream during the day, go for a gel formula. They're ultra light and will not cause make-up to run.

16. Don't be fooled into thinking your skin is protected all day if you apply a sunscreen. The sun protection factor (SPF) on sunscreen gives an indication of how long you can stay in the sun without burning. For example, if you normally burn in 10 minutes, wearing an SPF of 15 would protect you for 15 times longer. After the two-and-a-half hours, no additional amount of sunscreen will stop you from burning.

17. Clogged pores can be pimples waiting to happen. Purify your skin by dampening a clean hand towel with hot (not scalding) water and putting it over your face for about two minutes.

18. The face holds a lot of muscle tension and doesn't drain off toxins as quickly as the body, so if you are feeling tense and your complexion is drab, give your face a quick massage. With your fingertips, firmly press between your eyebrows and work up towards your hairline, then work along your cheekbone from your nose out to your ears.

19. Don't be frugal with a face mask. Spread it on as thickly as you would spread butter on bread. (That's if you're not dieting!)

20. Serums can be a real help to older skins that need more moisture. Apply them before moisturiser to heighten your skin's radiance.

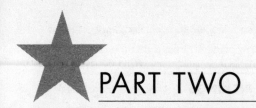

PART TWO

Mistake-proof makeovers to seduce the spotlight

When you're living your life in front of a long-lens camera, there are absolutely no short cuts to looking good. The reason why these stars seem to constantly shine brighter than a sparkling diamond is they're on a 24-hour party plan. It's the only way they can guarantee looking first class. Being famous means you not only have to look good for magazine covers, but every time you pop out for a pint of milk.

Celebrities know they should never look too off duty (dirty, unstyled hair is never a good Hollywood look) and even if resting (out of work) they're savvy enough to know they need to look the part of a star even if they haven't been called for an audition in over six months!

A celebrity's day will be bursting with appointments, so it's handy to have a *Smythson Health and Beauty Notes Book*, as bought by Gwyneth Paltrow, to keep track of one's essential indulgences. Even Jennifer Aniston's relaxed 'low-key' style takes more than five minutes. It's been rumoured that Jennifer is not averse to spending six hours being pampered from top to toe at day spas.

CELEBRITY PICKINGS *Smythson's of Bond Street are the world's stationers to the stars. The sought-after* Health and Beauty Notes Book *is a handbag-sized pink book that's indexed with such essentials as make-up, skincare, hair and nails. Under the chosen sections you can jot down your appointment and any treatment notes you wish to make.*

A well-organised beauty routine may sound frivolous but these appointments are crucial in maintaining the high standards that Hollywood has come to expect from its celebrities. Grey roots and chipped nails are the small details that the paparazzi will come down on like a ton of bricks. Stars need to look as though they've just stepped out of Selfridges' window display or straight off a magazine cover. This pays off by not only seducing the public with their 'beauty' but the movie directors too.

The very nature of celebrity as we know is all about looking glam-slam gorgeous and although some may say they were born with it, I say they work at it. Self-discipline is what makes a star.

'Creating a Hollywood image takes forethought and planning. A star, like a product, must have her own visual identity. Her make-up must reflect her personality or the personality she decides to show in public.'

Glauca Rossi, *veteran make-up artist to Meg Ryan, Bianca Jagger and Jerry Hall*

Never be fooled into thinking that celebrity beauty is all God-given. Even if they do claim it's down to dental floss, a slick of lip gloss or plenty of good sex with their latest Adonis, these influential style-setters go to a lot of effort to look effortless. And to help you radiate beauty greatness, I've begged, stolen and borrowed the best secrets – some of which celebrities would prefer to keep confidential – so you too can be a real scene-stealer.

One of the beauty secrets of wildly polished starlets is being in the know. Or employing people who know people in the know! Contacts are everything: when Gwyneth craves a bikini wax or Madonna needs a manicure, the most trusted beauty gurus in the field are called in at a minute's notice to deliver that million-dollar gloss. Collectively, these behind-the-scenes transformers are known as the star's 'dream team'. And take note: all-round beauticians are most definitely out. It's specialists that are in. 'Niche pampering' is the buzz term. So who are these style specialists?

The hip list: experts who can make all the difference

THE EYEBROW DESIGNER

If you thought great-looking eyebrows just grew, think again. Like everything in celebrity world, they are made to order. Eliza Petrescu is known as Queen of the Arch and is the founder of Eliza's Eyes, the first-ever boutique solely dedicated to the art of eyebrow shaping at the prestigious Avon Salon & Spa in Trump Tower, New York. The Wonder Woman of the perfect brow, Eliza's devotees include Jennifer Lopez, Oprah Winfrey and Natasha Richardson, who reveals, 'People tell me I have great eyebrows, and I correct them and say, "No, I have the greatest eyebrow designer!"' With accolades like this it's not surprising that Eliza's seven-minute makeover has been termed 'better than surgery'!

'Creating perfect eyebrows isn't just about trimming, plucking and tweezing,' Eliza says, 'it's about creating a look. A style. A feeling. It's about creating beauty. You wouldn't cut your own hair, so why would you try to shape your own eyebrows? The right eyebrow shape can really wake up your face and take years off. Eyebrows can change your look completely. They can make a face look sexy, intriguing, happy and polished – all with just a bit of subtle modification.'

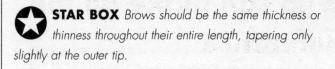

STAR BOX *Brows should be the same thickness or thinness throughout their entire length, tapering only slightly at the outer tip.*

Highbrow Ways to Shape Up:

Waxing: Just like body hair, brow hair can be waxed away in seconds. This is better than tweezing, as the hair grows back more slowly and finer.

Threading: A traditional Indian hair removal technique that has become increasingly sought after, threading involves using intricately twisted, specially strengthened cotton to lift hairs up from the root and quickly whip them out.

Plucking: For a quick do-it-yourself option, the tweezers can't be beaten. If you're uncertain about getting the right shape for your brows, see an expert who will shape them and then you can maintain the shape at home yourself.

Eliza's Can-do Tips for Achieving Perfect Brow Know-how

★ Place a pencil vertically at the side of your nose at the widest point of the base, so it extends over the inside corner of the eye and across the inner tip of the brow. Mark this point with a brow pencil. This is the most flattering place for your eyebrow to start.

★ Move the pencil so that it goes from the base of the nose to the outer corner of the eye and across the brow. Mark this point with a brow pencil. This should be the minimum length of your eyebrow, but it can be longer if you like.

★ From the base of the nose, move the pencil until it crosses the outer rim of the iris (the colour ring around the pupil) as you look ahead and intersect the brow. Mark this point with a brow pencil. This is ideally where the highest point of the arch should be.

★ Tweeze the hairs between the brows and under your natural brow for a clean silhouette.

★ When the space between the brows is clean and the space below the arch is shaped, start tweezing at the outer tip to find the length that is most becoming to you. But be careful not to tweeze beyond the mark for minimum brow length.

THE WAXER

Celebrities have to focus on the important things in life and that means keeping totally hair free, except on their head of course. Remember the uproar that Julia Roberts caused when she turned up at a film première waving hairy armpits? Such a Hollywood *faux pas*! Waxing under the arms, on the arms, legs, chin, nose and lips is on the roll call to obtain that all-over baby-smooth skin.

And the price of fame knows no modesty. The Brazilian bikini wax known in the business as a 'Gwyneth' is a celebrity must-have. Claimed as 'completely worth it' by its many devotees, including Jennifer Grey, Naomi Campbell and Kirsty Alley, the Brazilian wax, not to put too fine a point on it, takes it all away from the nether regions, leaving just a tiny strip of closely shorn hair in the front. It's referred to by oldtimers as an airstrip, a thong wax, Hollywood wax or a *Playboy* wax. In London the celebrity waxer of choice is Otylia Roberts and in New York it's the J Sisters (there are seven of them). In their busy salon they proudly display a signed picture of Gwyneth Paltrow with the message: 'To the Beloved J Sisters, you have changed my life!'

Things That Brazilian Waxing Virgins Need to Know

★ Don't look for a Brazilian waxer in the phone directory. The best way to find out about a good waxer is word of mouth.

★ All dignity will fly out of the window. Your waxer will know you as intimately as your gynaecologist.

You will be asked to strip down to nothing, spread your legs into all kinds of very embarrassing positions and have your bottom cheeks parted! Your best defence is to appear as though you think it's as normal as your waxer does.

★ It hurts. The most experienced waxers are the quickest. The ones who have to keep going over and over the same spot are to be avoided.

★ If the pain or indignity is too much to handle, look to laser hair removal. Laser light is absorbed by the dark pigment in the hair follicle, destroying it, but not the surrounding skin. Large areas of unwanted hair can be zapped quite quickly.

 STAR BOX *Half an hour before waxing, take a painkiller or a large shot of vodka!*

THE NAIL TECHNICIAN

Or manicurist to you and me. The nail technician is important. Celebrities know that the most noticeable nails are those that are unkempt.

The US-based celebrity manicurist simply known as Elle works wonders on the nails of Jennifer Lopez, Sandra Bullock and Isabella Rossellini. When asked which of her starry clients has the best nails, her reply is 'Sandra Bullock. She has the best long fingers with squoval [a cross between square and oval] nails – the strongest shape for natural nails.'

Quizzed on the three main troubleshooters known to

nailkind, Elle hails discoloured nails, white spots and peeling of the skin around the fingertips as the enemies. She says, 'Using dark-coloured polish without first applying a base coat is one of the reasons for discoloured nails. White spots are generally caused by a trauma to the nail and peeling of the skin can be caused by an allergic reaction to formaldehyde [always scan labels and avoid this harsh drying ingredient].'

★ **STAR BOX** *To achieve the classiest paint job, don't be frightened to use your polish. Have enough on the brush to work with and always roll the bottle backwards and forwards between your palms. Shaking it like a cocktail mixer encourages bubbles.*

Elle's Nail Principles

★ Every four weeks treat yourself to a manicure.

★ Every day, twice a day, apply hand cream.

★ Once a week file your nails and work on your cuticles. For filing, never file in a sawing direction, always file in one direction. For cuticles, always soak your fingers, then gently push your cuticles back with a cuticle stick.

★ Use an exfoliating sea salt scrub on the back of your hands. It instantly revitalises them.

Once Bitten . . .

Britney Spears has been flagged up more than once in paparazzi pictures with chewed nails. What's Elle's advice on serial nibblers? 'I ask them to leave one nail alone,' she says. 'Choose your pinkies, then ring finger and gradually work through the hand.' Focus on the appearance of the nail and surrounding skin and don't become obsessed with length.'

★ **STAR BOX** *If you're having a professional manicure, pay for it before, not after. Scratching around for payment can wreck the results.*

THE PEDICURIST

It's sandal season all year long for red-carpet troopers. And the vogue for thin-strapped sandals leaves no room for down-at-heel cracked heels. Fortunately, podiatrists (feet doctors) and pedicurists are on call to polish, pumice and pamper feet so they look hot to trot.

The secret to getting a celebrity foothold is in the preparation. A good and thorough pedicure can take as long as two hours. The feet are soaked, scraped, buffed, poked, pushed and painted. Then, just like a manicure, it's up to you to give them weekly TLC for heightened exposure.

First Steps to Fancy Feet

★ Massage your feet nightly, especially the heels, with an enriching cream to rid yourself of dry skin.

★ Use a pumice stone daily to gently rub your soles,

the balls of your feet and anywhere that is prone to callus build-up. Always get corns dealt with professionally.

★ Hairy toes are scary. When having your legs waxed, ask the therapist to whip off any hair on your feet too.

★ When painting, work from the little toe inwards to avoid smudging the fresh paint.

★ The shape of toenails should be square and just to the edge of your toe. Long looks crude and rounded off at the side can lead to in-growing toenails.

★ Replace emery boards regularly. An uneven grain causes uneven filing.

★ When painting toenails, always call upon the services of a toe separator. Toes are rarely straight and overlapping can cause smudging.

★ **STAR BOX** *Darker-coloured nail polishes help diminish imperfections by absorbing light and are easier to touch up. The more transparent you go, the better shape your toenails have to be in.*

How to look better naked

Every body has to be perfect when we're talking celebrity. Designers of front-plunging, back-skimming dresses have turned every bareable body part into a potential fashion hot spot. And if anyone knows how to buy a better-looking body and look good for their nude awakenings, plus feel ultra-confident at the same time, it's the stars.

TAN YOUR HIDE

There is a classic Californian saying: if you can't tone it, tan it! The definitive skin shade for the stars 365 days of the year is rich, sweet, honey brown. There's little doubt that a heavenly glow does wonders for the body. It evens up the smallest of imperfections (stretch marks, vitiligo and scar tissue), gives the illusion of improving skin tone – even on flabby thighs – and most importantly, makes us look slimmer. Celebrities fake it, of course, because they don't want their skin looking like leather by the time they hit 45. Even those with drool-worthy bodies rely on a self-tan's confidence-boosting magic.

Stars That Go for a Heavenly Glow

Jennifer Lopez, Victoria Beckham and Elizabeth Hurley all use tanners to make their skin look as though it's been giftwrapped in a lightly toasted body stocking.

★ Jennifer Lopez is a reputed devotee of the Fantasy Tan, a specially formulated airbrush system that applies a sunless, hassle-free, just-back-from-the beach tan in just 15 minutes.

★ Kylie Minogue prefers the St Tropez Express Bronze Treatment. With a formula of aloe vera leaf juice and AHA (fruit acid) it gives a streakless colour in just half an hour.

★ Jennifer Aniston is rumoured to love the Jean Paul Mist-On Tanning treatment where colour is applied by an automated misting process for an all-over golden tan.

★ Britney Spears has found a reason to fake it with Fake Bake. Voted the best self-tanner in a *New York Times* survey, it leaves skin looking sunkissed for up to seven days.

⭐ **STAR BOX** *Don't put tan on your feet at full strength. They are dryer than the other parts of the body and will absorb too much colour. Make a creamy lotion of both moisturiser and tan to custom blend.*

Fake It Easy

With self-tanning now as routine as applying mascara, it's imperative that limbs look genuinely golden with no telltale streaky marks in sight:

★ Exfoliate and moisturise first to ensure your body is baby-smooth soft.

★ Stained hands are a sure giveaway. Avoid this by wearing latex gloves.

★ Start tanning from your toes up.

★ When applying fake tan to the face, start in the centre and massage outwards. Make sure it doesn't collect around the nostrils, eyebrows and under the chin.

★ For a natural look, apply more fake tan to the places the sun catches first: the fronts of the legs and the shoulders. Use less around the knees, elbows, toes and fingers, but rub it in well.

★ Apply a small amount under the arms and breasts and around the bikini line.

★ Check your heels in the mirror and add a little more moisturiser to the creases in them after applying the lotion.

★ Allow at least 10 minutes for the tan to settle before dressing.

★ **STAR BOX** *If you've had a mishap with the application of your fake tan, apply whitening toothpaste to the bad spots to help it fade.*

THOROUGHBRED LEGS
Zapping Veins

When dresses slashed to the thigh and mini skirts are in, spider veins are definitely out. Veins can be the equivalent of a troublesome complexion and can otherwise blight a good pair of legs. As bare legs are *de rigueur* in celebrity land, a good pair of thick denier tights cannot be relied upon to hide any flaws.

A quick way to lose leg veins is by a procedure called microsclerotherapy. The secret of many a thoroughbred-looking leg, it involves injecting a small amount of saline solution designed to cause microscopic damage to the cells lining the vein. The body's repair mechanism then responds to this injury by trying to heal the vessel and in the process shrinks or obliterates it. Generally one injection is needed per vein or 'spray' of interconnecting veins. For two weeks after, the vessels may appear more prominent but will begin to fade after a week or so. There is no risk of scarring.

However, it's laser technology that is revolutionising treatment for zapping thread veins and none more so than the Lyra Laser System which is the first American FDA (Food and Drug Administration) cleared laser for all skin types. Known as the long-pulse laser, it selectively targets and destroys leg thread veins through a series of pulses of laser light. The longer wavelength penetrates deep within the leg and is attracted to the darker pigment in the veins, making it possible to treat a broad range of vessel sizes and depth, including deeper blue, purple and red blood vessels. The veins are destroyed by heat and the blood inside them coagulates and fades away.

It's also worth checking out the new creams that include vitamin K – a blood-clotting vitamin that plastic surgeons have used for years – and claim to diminish the appearance of thread veins.

★ **STAR BOX** *Follow on the heels of the best-dressed legs in the business and use leg shine for a sexy no-stocking look. Glide shimmer down the centre of thighs and shins to make them glisten and appear slimmer.*

In Search of Hair-free Legs

When it comes to fuzz-free legs, don't believe stars can be bothered with shaving and regular waxing. No, they look to the latest systems that promise permanent hair removal.

The Intense Pulse Light (IPL) system has had extraordinary results, even on dark skin which hasn't been suitable for treatment in the past because of its high melanin content. In simple terms: the IPL is attracted to the melanin in the hair and then converts to heat, destroying the follicle. Only hairs in the growing phase are destroyed, so several sessions are needed at monthly intervals.

So Long, Cellulite

Dimples can be cute on your chin, but not on your thighs or butt. Cellulite can be the great leveller in life. Jennifer Lopez, Naomi Campbell and Jerry Hall have all been unwittingly snapped with the dreaded puckering. According to research, 95 per cent of women suffer from cellulite, so if nothing else, it's one thing you've probably got in common with a celebrity!

'Cellulite is typically a female problem as fat cells on the lower part of the body store fat six times more readily than those on the upper body and release them six times less readily.'

Dr Elisabeth Dancey, *cellulite expert*

The orange-peel lumpy skin is caused by diet, water retention and poor circulation that cuts off blood flow to fat cells. When celebrities want to purge themselves of it, they ditch the caffeine, nicotine, saccharine and wine and switch to herbal tea and plenty of water.

They also look beyond creams to win the war on the orange-peel effect. A treatment called Endermologie is the only cellulite-reducing treatment to boast FDA approval. Imagine having a hand-held vacuum swept across your limbs, enthusiastically sucking up wobbly bits in the process, and you have an idea of what it involves.

Mesotherapy is another treatment that the stars swear by. This involves tiny injections of specific homoeopathic medicines just underneath the surface of the skin in the problem area. It's said to break down fat and improve circulation and lymphatic drainage.

★ **STAR BOX** *If the stars can't suck in their flaws, they have them sucked away by a new trendy injectable known as Lipo-dissolve. Shot directly into fat tissue, it melts away love handles and stubborn fat on the chin, hips, thighs, under the eyes and even on the knees.*

Get happy! In search of the great white smile

Forget the Versace dress and the Manolo heels, nothing draws the limelight like a megawatt smile. You know when there's a mega-bash on, as there's a rush on for teeth bleaching. For Oscar night, it's almost true to say that shades are worn to shield the eyes from the stars' blinding grins, as they know there's nothing like a full-fledged smile to warm cynical hearts and open (stage) doors.

Smiley happy people are more popular, appear more expressive and seem more flirtatious – even if they're not. The hiring of a good cosmetic dentist has to be up there with hiring a ruthless agent.

'Never underestimate the power of the smile. Your smile can work better than any make-up. Nowadays people turn to dentistry as a way of improving their appearance.'

Dr Phil Stemmer *of the Teeth for Life Clinic and dentist to Patsy Kensit, Sadie Frost and Jude Law*

It's easy to forget what an important role teeth play in your psychological state. Creating a healthy, natural and as-near-to-perfect smile as possible can alter your whole perception of yourself and dramatically increase your self-confidence. And you're never too old to improve on your smile. Tom Cruise had a brace fitted well out of his twenties, *Armageddon* director Michael Bay so desperately wanted Ben Affleck to star in the film that he paid to have the actor's tiny teeth capped and pop princess Kylie Minogue's smile was made bigger by closing gaps in her teeth and correcting her bite.

STEPS TO SMILING LIKE A STAR
Teeth Whitening

> 'Everyone wants whiter teeth because it makes us look healthier and younger. Close encounters with major stainers such as tea, coffee and nicotine are going to take their toll on your smile sooner or later.'
>
> **Dr Sunny Luthra,** *leading dentist at Capital Dental, who guarantees the dazzle factor for many a television star*

Some people also suffer staining caused by antibiotics or minute cracks in the teeth that take up stain and affect the colour. 'But be advised that whitening can only lighten your existing tooth colour and only works on natural teeth,' Dr Luthra divulges. 'It will not work on crowns or veneers.'

So how does this procedure work? It's simple, if not glamorous. A plastic retractor is put in the mouth to hold the cheeks and tongue out of the way and a rubber coating is applied to gums to protect them. A special solution containing hydrogen peroxide is then painted onto the teeth. A laser light then activates the solution, making the whitening process fast and easy. The end result is brighter, whiter teeth you'll want to grin and bare. And one thing celebrities remember is: the bigger the smile, the bigger the bucks!

★ **STAR BOX** *Wear silver jewellery as opposed to gold near the face. The yellow tone in gold accentuates the yellow in teeth. This makes for a great excuse to wear diamonds.*

Veneers

Most dental cosmetic improvements are achieved by using porcelain veneers that enable a smile to be corrected aesthetically without compromising the long-term health of the teeth. It's like having false fingernails fitted over the front of the teeth. Classed as the *couture* of dental work, veneers can hide a multitude of sins, from chipped or discoloured teeth to crooked teeth and gaps. Originally developed in the 1930s for Hollywood movie stars, they are still a favourite with celebrities today. Many stars, such as Catherine Zeta Jones, have had them to make their smiles fuller and straighter.

Cosmetic Fillings

Unsurprisingly, most celebrities don't want to show a mouth full of silver fillings when they open their mouths to laugh. Not only can it look ugly, but it can also give away their age! The procedure for cosmetic fillings is straightforward: old amalgam or decay is removed, the hole is shaped and filled with a tooth-coloured paste or composite. The composite is moulded in the tooth then set hard with ultraviolet light, making fillings virtually invisible.

Electro-surgery

Many celebrities' primary objective is straight-looking white teeth. And that nice even smile can't shine if the gums are covering the teeth. Electro-surgery works by applying a fine electric current to the gums to remove one cell at a time. Gums are then pushed back so more teeth are on show. Just think of it as pushing the cuticles back on nails. This simple and painless procedure can be used to help lengthen the appearance of teeth, reduce a gummy smile and ensure that the gums form a harmonious shape around the teeth. Gums should ideally be crescent-shaped, with the gumline mirroring the top lip line.

★ **STAR BOX** *Avoid food or drink that would stain a white shirt – they'll do the same for your teeth. No wonder celebrities hail grilled chicken and champagne as their mainstays!*

Eye openers, lip slicks and other must-have make-up tricks

The idea for this section is not to give you a master-class step-by-step make-up lesson, but to inform you of the beauty élite's secrets that can really, really make a difference. These are tips that every expert knows, but never lets out of the bag. They will really enhance your big-night-out beauty look – and they don't take hours either.

'When you're in a hurry, stick to what you know with colours and products. Opt for a sheer lipstick that requires less precision than those with pigment and can be applied on the move without a mirror.'

Sharon Dowsett, *make-up artist to Renée Zellweger and Hilary Swank*

MAKING THE GREATEST OF FACES

But fast-tracking your beauty routine is of little use if you don't know how to apply make-up to enhance and flatter. Valentine Gotti-Alexander, a Paris-based make-up artist who boasts a movie background and has worked with stars such as Sigourney Weaver, Juliette Binoche and Catherine Deneuve, advocates getting to know your face – intimately. 'So many people apply their make-up in such a deadpan way the end result can be that of wearing a mask,' she says. 'Some celebrities are not necessarily beautiful in the conventional sense, but they seem beautiful as they put the light back into their face, give off an aura with the right make-up and know the correct colour to use for their skin. They embellish their look.'

Valentine runs Face Focus sessions at London's celebrity hang-out hotel The Sanderson and for an hour and a half divulges her movie make-up tips. Unique in her approach, she gets her clients to pull various faces:

★ The Fish Face: 'Suck the cheeks in and the high and low cheekbones you never knew you had pop out and you can then play them up,' she says.

★ Likewise with the Mona Lisa smile. 'It brings the apples of the cheeks into sharp focus,' Valentine says.

★ The Marilyn Monroe Pout: 'So many times women look into the mirror stony-faced to apply make-up and they never see their complete facial form,' reveals Valentine. Practise kissing your reflection and you'll get an idea of your lips' natural shape. And as for the complexion, 'Unless you can afford to have a lighting technician follow you around to give off that movie-star soft-lit glow, avoid fluorescent light: it steals away all colour. For dinner always, always choose candlelit restaurants!'

THE BEAUTY SECRETS OF THE RED-CARPET ELITE

High-wattage make-up is just as important as the gown and the hair when a star wants to shine. The looks, the talent, the gorgeous husband and the Hollywood connections may well make for success, but if her chosen lipstick shade makes her complexion look faded, she won't radiate.

Jeanine Lobell is New York's top make-up artist and creator of Stila Cosmetics. Diane Lane, Julianne Moore, Cate Blanchett and Cameron Diaz all have her telephone number. Jeanine's trademark is sexy, understated make-up. 'My main goal,' she says, 'is to always make a woman look and feel pretty. Some stars love shimmer, others colour and some feel more comfortable wearing neutral tones, but whatever they're into I have one rule: play up one focal feature, otherwise you'll look over made-up. Concentrating on either the eyes or the mouth is what can really make a face pop.'

Although regularly waving her mascara wand on the night for Academy Award nominees, for everyday make-up, Jeanine advocates just using powder if you have great skin, an eyelash curler which works as an 'instant wake-up call', a shiny lip gloss, blusher and a mascara that leaves lashes 'soft and fuzzy', not stiff and hard.

Jeanine's Fabulous Five Hollywood Make-up Tricks

1. Paint mascara on the lower lashes with a brush rather than with the mascara wand. This gives a better impact and frames the eyes with a lush lash-line.

2. Apply a soft-coloured shimmer shadow in the inner corner 'V' area of the eye. This will give eyes a brighter, more sparkly effect.

3. For an easy eye look, colourwash the lid with a light beige shadow. Choose from shimmery or matt.

4. Don't put foundation all over your face, only on areas that need it. This will make your complexion look natural and not so made-up.

5. Place some rosy nude shimmer cream in the middle of both upper and lower lip. Blend to give the illusion of a fuller mouth. Then take shimmer powder and highlight the cheekbones, above browbone and under the jawline. This will bring light to the face.

'When you need to glam it up, think about make-up that makes you look like yourself at your most gorgeous. The looks you see on the red carpet are great inspiration, but they can be hard to pull off in real life. Make them work for you by creating toned-down versions. If you love the idea of blue, green or purple eye shadow, just try lining the upper lashline only in navy or amethyst.'

Bobbi Brown, *make-up artist to Minnie Driver and Alicia Silverstone*

ARE YOU WEARING YESTERDAY'S FACE?

Has your make-up routine become just that? Are you still wearing blue eyeliner and matt foundation that's three shades deeper than your skintone? If so, then it's time to dig yourself out of that great big beauty rut. Think of Madonna, Sharon Stone and Nicole Kidman – all confident and attractive women that constantly update their look so their image stays fresh. Do you think they would have been so successful if they had kept their look from 1989?

The women that often find themselves looking dated are ones that usually have limited time and find themselves going back to their 'comfort range' of tried and tested favourites. However, what you may view as timeless, others regard as outdated. So what can you do? As we know, A-listers have an army of make-up artists on call, but you too can create a new you without too much hassle or expense.

First off decide whether you are in a rut. Do you follow the same basic make-up routine regardless of the occasion or what you're wearing? Have you worn the same colours for the past couple of years or more? Have you noticed that your favourite lip or eye colour has had a renaissance from the 70s? If the answers are 'Yes, yes, yes', your look is living in the past.

Rarely is there need to invest in a whole new make-up bag. There's nothing wrong with keeping a few things from your own comfort range, but the secret is adding additional colour so it never looks tired. The key is checking out new formulations (the dry look of wearing in triplicate: opaque lipstick, ultra matt eye shadow and ultra matt foundation is so over) and not shying away from new seasonal colours. They're there to enjoy wearing. As make-up becomes more experimental, it's all too easy to take one look at it and write it off. But the art is to take the effect and water it down to suit your style. Warm yourself to the idea of new colour by sticking with an old favourite – say a brown eyeshadow – and then adding an additional colour you wouldn't normally go for.

Mistakes That Make-up Losers Make

Lipstick on the teeth. Always do a smile check in the mirror before facing your public.

Racing stripes on cheeks. The little brushes that come with blush are always too small. They make stripes. Use a big soft brush to apply powder and your fingertips for creams and gels.

Raccoon eyes. Most women are fooled into thinking that a very light concealer will cover dark circles. They never will. A yellow undertone concealer will look natural.

Clown mouths. Remember, a dark lipliner married with a light lipstick is never acceptable.

Over-tweezed brows. These are usually seen as a desire for total control, a trait people often associate with someone who is obsessive and neurotic!

Clumpy lashes. Adding more mascara does not guarantee fuller lashes, just a mess.

Matching make-up to clothing. No, no, no!

Remember darker colours only minimise lips. Never be tricked into lining outside the natural lipline. You won't look like Angelina Jolie, only like The Joker.

SSSHH! 20 GET-GORGEOUS TIPS FOR INSTANT GLAMOUR

'Glamour', 'polish' and 'A-list sophistication' are the buzz words when I'm talking red-carpet beauty. Celebrities are constantly updating their look because their status has bought them the privilege of enjoying the expertise of the most creative and talented make-up artists in the world. Now you too can learn the tricks that keep them looking gorgeous with these true insider secrets from the mavericks of make-up:

1. Red-carpet queens Nicole Kidman, Renée Zellweger and Penelope Cruz all love slicking their lips with red for a touch of old Hollywood glamour, looking hot, sexy, fearless and fresh. Wear this with little other make-up. Red lips against a bare skin with a lightly defined eye looks striking.

2. For after-hours skin that literally sparkles in front of the camera Jeanine Lobell lets on that she mixes a tiny bit of loose pearlised beige eyeshadow into foundation before smoothing it on.

3. For thicker-looking lashes without clumping, make-up artist Laura Mercier, who is called upon by Madonna, Susan Sarandon, Sarah Jessica Parker and Mariah Carey, explains, 'It's not what you apply, but the way in which you apply it. Take the mascara wand and wiggle it on the root of the lashes.'

4. If your complexion craves a little powder to keep make-up from sliding, Mercier explains, 'When using a brush to apply loose powder, use the side of a powder brush, not the top. This will help to distribute

the powder lightly and evenly, instead of it going on in an uneven clump.'

5. If there's one colour that makes almost every woman look as sweet as candy, it's hot pink. A staple look for Sarah Jessica Parker and Kate Hudson is mixing pale skin with a soft, glossy pink lip and soft eyes. The only pink that doesn't flatter is a frosted pale one.

6. A smoky eye does not equal a black eye! Karen Kawahara, a Hollywood make-up artist who creates Salma Hayek's radiant looks, reveals, 'For a great Oscar look I love adding drama to the eyes. I use greys, browns or midnight blues instead of black, which can look harsh. I apply the colour around the eyelashes and then smudge it out and blend it up into the brow-bone.'

7. Jennifer Lopez is one diva who doesn't shy away from punchy colour. Witness her wearing sea-green eye make-up. The rule: pick one shade (only) and colour-wash over the entire eyelid for great effect.

8. Many a make-up artist knows that injecting a fresh radiance to the skin is down to smart products. Luminising make-up boosts luminosity. The law is to pick products that contain a hint of pearl or shimmer. Never glitter. And never overdo a good thing. If you use shimmer shades on your eyes and cheeks, then keep your base matt.

9. Thought Kylie Minogue's, Nicole Kidman's and Jennifer Lopez's eyelashes were that thick? You have to be kidding. They know that fake lashes can juice up eyes at night. Either place a couple of individual lashes

in the outer corners of each eye for a come-hither look, or at 10 and 2 o'clock over the irises for a more open look.

10. Talking about lash acts, invest in a pair of eyelash curlers. Every star knows that clamping their eyelashes in a steel trap is worth the effort for an open-eyed look. Always curl before applying mascara, otherwise the lashes will be too brittle and might break. If you're time-starved, you could always get your lashes permed. Yes, really! The effect lasts for up to six weeks.

11. Bronzers are a great automatic wake-up call for the complexion. Bronze gives the look of sun under the skin – really vibrant and healthy. But too much and you can resemble a pumpkin. Select a shade that's only two shades darker than your natural colouring. To avoid looking roasted, limit the rest of your make-up to mascara and just a dab of sheer lip gloss.

12. Forget eye jobs and fancy creams. To deflate under-eye puffiness, put two teaspoons in the freezer for five minutes. Balance the bottom of the spoons on the area beneath your eyes and see the difference.

13. Before applying a dark lipstick, smooth on some lip balm then run a damp, warm flannel gently back and forth across your lips to whip away any dead skin. 'I do it all the time before a singer or actress goes on set,' says make-up artist Daniel Sandler. 'If lips look cracked, so will the lipstick.'

14. Forget liquid liner unless you're committed to hours of practice. Use kohl instead. Line the inner rim of the eye to add definition without heaviness and never be

tempted to smudge black kohl low under the eyes. It won't make you look steamy, just hungover and tired.

15. An A-list seductress knows that to play up cheekbones you need to highlight them. 'Feel your cheekbones with your fingers and highlight the top with a pearlised highlighter,' says Sharon Dowsett.

16. To give skin a 'poreless' finish, stroke foundation, powder and blusher downwards. Why? Because otherwise you'll be pushing pigment up and into your pores and so highlighting them.

17. Ever seen a lip shade on a star but been unable to find it at the cosmetics counter? That's because a make-up artist is, well, an artist and uses a palette full of colours to blend personal shades. Buy five lipsticks: one true pink, one deep brown, one clear orange, one absolute red and one pale and translucent. Mash them into a compartmentalised paint box and you can whip up dozens of new lipstick colours.

18. 'For ridiculously white eyes,' says Sharon Dowsett, 'use eye drops sparingly. Black is the most contrasting colour to white, so outline the eye with black kohl and use lashings of black mascara. It worked for Cleopatra!' For baby blondes, brown mascara works best, otherwise you'll wind up looking like Barbie.

19. Make up in the hardest and most unflattering light. Think flashgun, facing-the-cameras scenario. If you look good there, you'll look great anywhere

20. To prevent clumpy lashes, wipe your mascara brush with a tissue before you use it. You may think you're wasting it, but your lashes will look gorgeous. To make

up for it when you've finished a tube of mascara, recycle the brush. Wash it and use the wand as an eyelash brush.

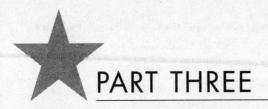

PART THREE

Oscar-worthy hair and how to get it

When it comes to stealing the spotlight, style gurus may well preach about each season's latest fashion must-have, whether it's a breathtaking bag costing a month's rent or Manolo heels to die for, but ask them what single investment will update and revitalise your image in a nanosecond and the answer will always be the right hair. For right now. And it doesn't matter how radiant your skin looks, what designer clothes are hanging off your back or how big and shiny your rocks, if your hair's not looking the way you want it to look, you actually don't feel good. It's deeply psychological!

Look through the celebrity archive and you'll notice that even some of the most beautiful and photographed women have had their fair share of hair blunders. But once they've hit upon the right stylist, colourist and hair products, their mane begins to look far from lame and starts looking fabulous. And that's where you can take your hair cue for a better-looking do. With the right cut, colour and use of 'prescriptive' products, your hair can be a huge asset, just like that of any major Hollywood player. A good cut can soften your features, while the correct use of colour can bring your skin tone alive, give your eyes more vibrancy, downplay bad features and highlight good ones. And the intelligent use of products can instantly double your hair's sex appeal.

Here we get to the roots of how to get great, seductive, Oscar-winning hair.

★ **STAR BOX** *Oscar-winning hair takes time and effort. And plenty of it. A Pantene Pro-V study concluded that we spend 22 minutes a day styling our hair. Avoid bad hair days by getting up half an hour earlier.*

Shear genius: your best cut ever

Haircuts can be so important that some of them have even taken on a life of their own. Farrah Fawcett was one angel who inspired many a flicked-out look. Another influential style was the Purdy haircut created by John Frieda for Joanna Lumley in her *Avengers* role.

> 'The Purdy cut was simply inspired by looking at Joanna Lumley's face shape and adding a boyish element which she made extremely feminine. The phenomenon took off because when I cut it, I realised it was something different and Joanna looked incredibly beautiful.'
>
> **John Frieda**, *celebrity hairdresser*

Fast-forward a couple of decades or so and we've had the Meg and the Rachel. Meg Ryan and Jennifer Aniston are as famous for their hair as they are for their flair. Ryan dumped her frumpy, frizzed-out do along with her hot rollers and turned to top stylist and her secret hair weapon, Sally Hershberger at John Frieda, for a new edgy style.

'I couldn't predict the long-lasting impact and interest in the "shag", but it seemed that the haircut happened in tandem with Meg's profile really taking off.'

Sally Hershberger, *stylist to Meg Ryan*

To make an entry on the best-tressed list, celebrities have to leave their egos at the door and put their look in the hands of the stylist. You do too. It's safe to hang onto the style you had five years ago, but ask yourself: would your average Hollywood hotshot be as sizzling as she is today if she had stayed stuck in a hairstyle rut? We don't think so. Nicole Kidman, Jennifer Aniston and Sarah Jessica Parker have all shown themselves to be style chameleons when we're talking hair.

Your relationship with your hairstylist can be one of the most rewarding beauty experiences, so much so they can become your NBF (new best friend). Just ask leading hair-stylist Charles Worthington, who teases the tresses of Rosanna Arquette and Joely Richardson and counts many of his celebrity clients as more than just his 2 o'clock appointment, or session hairstylist James Brown, who is Kate Moss's mane man and has literally landed her plum advertising campaigns with his hair vision. Brown is also part of her 'in-crowd' posse too.

'The foundation to any good style is the cut. Anything else that follows is purely cosmetic.'

Trevor Sorbie, *international hairstylist*

And this is the no-big-secret of a head-turning style. A savvy stylist will simply adapt the various well-engineered cuts worn by celebrities to suit your hair texture and the shape of your face to give style, form and that all-exclusive wow factor.

THE 10 COMMANDMENTS FOR A GREAT HAIRCUT

1. Be nosy. Personal recommendations are always helpful when it comes to looking for a talented snipper. If you see someone whose hair inspires you, ask where they've had it done.

2. Check out the salon carefully. Look at the clientèle and tune into the general vibe of the place. They way the stylists dress, the music they play, for example. These all offer clues as to whether it's the right place for you. When booking your consultation, bear in mind stylists have personal strengths, regardless of their level of experience. So if you have curly hair, for example, mention it over the phone.

3. Have a frank talk with your stylist along with a thorough consultation before getting a cut. It's free and you can see whether or not you connect with the stylist. He should ask you questions about how your hair behaves, how much time you have to spend on your hair and how you see your personality.

4. Don't be scissor shy. Don't rule out a style because you think your hair can't carry it off. You'd be surprised at what can work.

5. Take picture backup. It cuts to the chase and can

ultimately help your stylist deliver a great cut. Don't feel embarrassed whipping out a picture of Sharon Stone. Your stylist knows you're not thinking you look like her, you just crave her hair!

6. Avoid impulse cuts at all costs – they rarely work. Splitting up with your boyfriend is not a reason to go from brunette to blonde or from long to short. It's the time for your heart to get emotional, not your hair!

7. Cut before you colour. Pre-cut colour can look random, or worse, fight the new cut. Get the haircut first and then have the colour done.

8. Make a date with your stylist every eight to 12 weeks. If your stylist is A-list worthy, he'll be booked solid. So book him now and don't wait until your hair looks desperate.

9. Insist on a style with options. With the exception of short hair, you should be able to put it up, blow it out, change the parting and do a number of different looks. That's the secret of 'international' hair.

10. If you're not happy with your cut, speak up. Most top salons have re-do policies. Likewise, if the cut isn't working after a week, call and ask for a (free) re-adjustment cut.

HAIR RE-DO – FOR WHEN YOU'RE TEMPTED TO TRY A WHOLE NEW STYLE

Ever looked in the mirror and realised you're well and firmly stuck in a hair timewarp? There are plenty of celebrities out there who've had the same style for years – whether it suits them or not – and guesses are their careers have stood still as well. Sometimes it can be hard to move on, but if you feel that your hairstyle falls between stamp collecting and trainspotting on the excitement scale, maybe your inner Madonna is telling you to spin doctor your look and try out a whole new style.

10 Excuses to Transform your Hair

1. You Crave a Full-on Hair Affair

'There's no better way to give your self-esteem a boost than changing your hair,' reveals Charles Worthington. 'It's the quickest way to rock your image. A new style – especially if it's radically different – signals to everyone else that they should look at you with new eyes.'

2. A Stunning Dress Demands a New Do

A jaw-dropping dress simply asks for Oscar-winning hair. Even if you don't fancy going for the chop, rising to the occasion is always a hot Hollywood look. Swooped-up Audrey Hepburn style adds a *haute* new twist to evening dressing. Just ask Julia Roberts and Nicole Kidman.

3. You're Beyond Long Hair

Getting sick of your long hair? You're in good company. At one time or another Kate Winslet, Cate Blanchett, Liv Tyler and Penelope Cruz have all gone for the snip. Short hair is sharp and means business. But go for the chop when you're feeling good about yourself.

4. You're Fed Up with In-between Hair

Hair that's neither short nor long can drive you style crazy. The answer? Extensions. Mermaid-style hair can get you past the in-between stage of hair and give you Rapunzel-like tresses until your own have grown. Victoria Beckham, Cameron Diaz and Pamela Anderson have all faked longer hair.

5. **You've Just Had a Mini Me**

Having a baby can be a catalyst for change, including your hair. But be warned: don't go for drastic changes when feeling hormonal. And yes, that includes PMS! If the whim takes you, start off making subtle changes and when you're feeling stronger you can evolve your look.

6. **You're Getting Hitched**

There's no better motive to revamp your do than for your wedding day, but military-style planning is essential. Book several appointments before your nuptials so that you can try out different ways of styling your hair and wearing your headdress. Celebrities spend months before their big day consulting their stylist. When serial bride Jennifer Lopez married her now ex-husband Cris Judd, she flew out a top stylist from New York to California.

7. **You Want to Upstage Your Ex's New Squeeze**

Nicole Kidman went blonde when Tom Cruise fell into the arms of Penelope Cruz and stole the moment. Break-ups are one of the major reasons that women change their hair, but a long chat with your stylist is called for at this time. You don't want it to be something you're going to regret.

8. **You're Seeing the First Strands of Grey**

Mother Nature can be cruel. Just when you're feeling confident about how to wear your hair, she peppers it with a smattering of grey! Colourist Jo Hansford has the answers. 'Up to 20 per cent of grey, I tend to recommend a vegetable or semi-permanent colour for hair. This will enhance or give depth to the hair, as well as overtone the natural colour. If a lighter or warm colour is chosen above the natural hair colour, then the grey hair will take on a lowlight effect.'

9. **You've Shed a Lot of Weight**

When pounds melt away, your figure isn't the only thing to change. The shape of your face does too and that means reanalysing your style. Losing weight can emphasise your bone structure more, so now is the time to seek advice from your hair guru.

10. **You've Just Turned 30**

Half of the sexiest female celebrities are aged over 30. The moral of this tale? Celebrities know age is only a number and don't let it stop them from becoming hair-inspired. Hair can instantly de-age you if you know what cut and colour suits: you can leave the salon with the confidence of a 30-year-old and the looks of a 25-year-old.

★ STAR BOX *As well as your face shape, consider your features too. Let's be brutal: short hair reveals everything about you. Those with a prominent nose or sticky-out ears always need a little more hair.*

TAKING THE PLUNGE

So you've examined, consulted, mulled, devised and bitten your nails over going for a completely new you. You're fully aware that there is no way to uncut hair once it's lying on the salon floor and you understand that a new injection of bold and bright colour may mean adjusting to a new hair texture and new make-up. Tell yourself you are willing to learn what it takes to keep your hair looking A-list. Just make sure your transformer (stylist) explains the how-tos as he goes along. And that means, for you, not burying your head in a magazine at the salon, but taking note of how he styles your hair and what products he plays your hair up with.

Facing Up to the Best Cut for Your Face

Seeking out a smart cut that plays up everything you love about your face and downplays everything you don't is crucial for A-list hair confidence.

If Your Face is Square

Celebrity inspiration: Sandra Bullock
The goal: To soften the angles of your chin and forehead.
Go for: Sexy waves to take the edge off a square face. This sophisticated look will help soften sharp angles and harsh jawlines. Heaps of volume at the top and soft, feathered layers around the face will also divert attention from a square jawline. If the style lies flat to the head it can accentuate squareness. Break up the shape using light styling products.

Stay away from: Bobs that end above or by your ears. Long, layer-free hair can wind up making your face look boxy.

If Your Face is Round

Celebrity inspiration: Renée Zellweger
The goal: To elongate and slim down your face.
Go for: Longer pieces that fall onto the face to give the illusion that your cheeks are slimmer and more structured. A graduated bob cut onto the face and high at the back looks great, as does a shoulder-grazing do with blunt ends that gives the illusion of lengthening the face.
Stay away from: Structured cuts that can look too severe and emphasise the width of the face.

If Your Face is Long

Celebrity inspiration: Jennifer Aniston
The goal: To minimise your face length.
Go for: A shorter style – but not above the bottom of your chin so your hair looks thicker and your face wider. The quickest and easiest way of minimising face length is with a fringe. Disguise a long forehead with a thick blunt fringe – you'll be surprised how feminine it looks.
Stay away from: Long straight hair with no graduation or layers. It will look like a pair of curtains and give the illusion of pulling your face down even further.

If your Face is Oval

Celebrity inspiration: Sharon Stone

The goal: Anything that takes more time than you have to style.

Go for: Almost any style works with this face shape. Simply work with other features of your face to create the right style. A bob that kicks out at the end gives volume around the bottom of the face, whereas smooth waves parted on the side will detract from a small chin and break up harsh symmetry.

Stay away from: Too much height to the crown, especially with a short fringe. It can make a small oval face look smaller.

If your Face is Heart-shaped

Celebrity inspiration: Drew Barrymore

The goal: To make your forehead look less broad and inject fullness into the bottom half of your face.

Go for: Soft layers to soften your chin area. Keep the layers cut as close to your jawline as possible so that they can fall seductively onto your face. If your hair is curly, try a chin-length cut with slightly uneven ends.

Stay away from: Super-short super-shorn cuts.

Triple your hair's sex appeal

What is the 'X' factor that makes one woman's hairstyle sexy and another look as though she should be working in a library? Some celebrities have hair that looks as though they've just rolled out of their satin-sheeted bed after a night of love – ruffled, tousled and downright dirty-looking!

Then there's the art of hairplay: twiddling it, flicking it and wrapping it around your finger all signal you're confident and direct and willing to play the game. From Lady Godiva to a modern billboard star, hair has long had the power to entice, tantalise and tease. Hair is a secondary female sexual characteristic and changing its colour and length is claimed to make us more desirable. But perhaps the greatest quality about hair is that you can change it and work it to get what or who you want. All you need to know is how to package and style it for full-scale seduction:

Start by paying some attention to your hair, rather than just bunging it up in a ponytail and forgetting about it.

Think what you want your hair to say about you and then style accordingly.

Play up the hair-over-the-eye trick. Elizabeth Hurley knows how to work this so well! A long asymmetrical fringe or a low side parting obscures one eye so you come over all mysterious.

> ★ **STAR BOX** *Nonchalantly pulling your hair up off your neck and piling it up on your head then letting it fall again can be the metaphorical equivalent of lifting up and taking down your clothes!*

SEXY FRINGE BENEFITS

Seduction hair can simply mean adding a fringe. Here's how to choose the right style for your face.

Long and Layered: Layered fringes are the most versatile and probably the sexiest as, like Elizabeth Hurley, you can lower your eyes and flirt behind them. They work on any face shape – even round – and won't overwhelm a small forehead.

Short and Wispy: Fringes are often the finishing touch on a cropped cut. Think Mia Farrow circa 1960s. They look best on small urchin-like faces. The way they frame the face makes them a great option for those who want fringes that draw lots of attention to their eyes.

Thick and Heavy: Fringes like these tend to call attention to the centre of the face. They make a strong statement on almost anyone, but are particularly good at camouflaging a long face, making it look smaller. Those with wide faces should have some shape to their fringe, avoiding styles cut straight across the forehead.

> ⭐ **STAR BOX** *If going for a fringe you need to make your eyebrows more defined, otherwise they can't be seen through the hair. If your brows are sparse, fill them in with a darker brown eyeshadow.*

How to do high-performance Hollywood colour

Celebrity stylists may well grab all the headlines, but it's the colourists who wield the real power at the salon. They alone can make your skin look more luminous, your eyes brighter and your crowning glory just that: thicker, richer and shinier. The message is clear: 'Long live colour!' These days every VIP star has their colourist on speed dial along with their yoga teacher and manicurist. Why? Because they know a trade of shade can spin them a fresh new look in less time than it takes to choose a designer dress. Bingeing with colour is fun, as Nicole Kidman knows. Nicole can always cut it as a redhead, but she flirts with being a born-again blonde. This is one woman who uses her hair colour to get herself noticed. But what's the difference between a good hue and a brilliant one?

'You always know when you've got someone's hair colour absolutely perfect, as it complements the eyes, skin tone and the season.'

Brad Johns, *artistic director at the Avon Salon & Spa in New York, colourist to Natasha Richardson and Christy Turlington*

Brad has pioneered every look from chunky highlights to the buttery blonde and maintains the most lustworthy colour is the one you possessed as a child. 'The most brilliant colour is that of a child on the beach. The hair's natural highlights and vibrancy are my inspiration,' he states.

The secret for going all out for colour is not to shy away from brave new hues. Celebrities that gather to the spotlight like bees to a honey pot have realised that a few subtle streaks just won't do. They've wised up that colour can be changed and adapted pretty quickly and with this in mind, there are generally far fewer rules to follow in regard to suitability for colour. Colour supremo Jo Hansford, who tends to the colour of Cate Blanchett and Angelina Jolie in her Mayfair salon, agrees: 'Everyone knows that a great new style can make you feel a million dollars, but add colour to the mix and you can experience a total emotional turnaround. I've seen people walk out the salon instantly upbeat and tell me they feel more glamorous.'

'The rule books have always said that you should consider your complexion and the shade of your eyes when choosing a hair colour. The rule books are there to be broken. Try telling Debbie Harry that she didn't look good as a blonde!'

Nicky Clarke, *celebrity hairstylist*

THE BUZZ OF BLONDE

Blonde and ambitious: Madonna, Sarah Jessica Parker, Gwyneth Paltrow, Kate Hudson, Renée Zellweger

Blonde because you're: Sexy, dizzy, playful, optimistic, communicative

When to go for blonde: If you have blue eyes and a medium to light complexion, blonde hair would probably suit you. Otherwise choose golds, coppers and honey-coloured highlights that add lightness and movement and require less upkeep. Jo Hansford suggests a light creamy blonde for a very pale, flawless complexion or, for those with pink skin tone, honey blonde. For those with brown eyes and neutral skin tones, choose copper blonde to enliven a sallow skin tone or pale complexion. Ash blonde works for blue-eyed beauties whose skin is not too pale.

Who shouldn't go there? Redheads can have problems going blonde as the red pigment can result in a brassy effect, especially if trying to go too light. There are also several issues that can arise when going from dark to blonde. 'Stick to softer blondes rather than an ash blonde,' says Hansford.

★ **STAR BOX** *As a brunette Cameron Diaz doesn't take centre stage. As a blonde she shakes off the girl-next-door image and morphs into a screen goddess.*

BRAVO FOR BRUNETTES

A darker shade of pale: Julia Roberts, Elizabeth Hurley, Sandra Bullock, Catherine Zeta Jones

Brunette because you're: Earthy, natural, genuine, reliable, serious, sultry

When to go brunette: 'Celebrities have wised up to the fact that you don't have to be blonde to bag a starring role in a film,' says Hansford. 'The advantages to being a brunette are there are no root regrowth problems and more scope on the colour front. A brunette can be a whole range of colours and these can be dabbled with as often as you want.' While black hair can be too much, a dark brunette can look quite stunning. There can be nothing more frustrating for some colourists than seeing a 'virgin' brunette. Many a celeb (Liz Hurley, Catherine Zeta Jones and the late Audrey Hepburn included) have had their colourist liven up their shade with sparks of lighter colour, usually at the front of the hair, to give an alluring appeal while lifting too-solid tones and adding depth.

Who shouldn't go there? If your complexion is too fair going brunette can simply draw away all colour, making your features look quite definite.

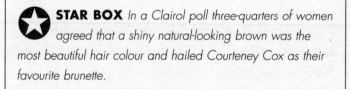

STAR BOX *In a Clairol poll three-quarters of women agreed that a shiny natural-looking brown was the most beautiful hair colour and hailed Courteney Cox as their favourite brunette.*

GET AHEAD WITH RED

Red and hot: Julianne Moore, Nicole Kidman (sometimes), Cynthia Nixon, Gillian Anderson

Red because you're: Fiery, intense, passionate, impulsive

When to go red: What redhead doesn't walk into a room and swivel heads? Red is a colour that demands to be noticed. If you have fair skin you can handle anything from a strawberry blonde to the more vibrant reds, whereas dark and olive skin look best with auburn and burgundy shades. Celebrity international colourist Daniel Galvin is a lover of rich copper reds. He explains, 'These are best on pinky skin tones, as this colour infuses hair with a vibrant shine, bringing green and hazel eyes into clear focus.'

Who shouldn't go there? 'Avoid red if you have a pink-based skin tone or dark features such as eyebrows or eyes,' divulges Jo Hansford. 'Also, if you have no natural red pigment, going red can be hard. Red molecules are the longest of artificial pigments, so they are the last to go in and the first to come out.'

 STAR BOX *For those that want to flirt with red but feel a little colour shy, opt for chestnut and maroon. These are more wearable colours.*

I Love Hue! Your at-a-Glance Colour Guide

If you have: Gold, strawberry blonde or warm brown hair, fair peach-toned skin, blue eyes
Cue your hue: Creamy and honey blonde, copper and russet reds

If you have: Ash blonde, mouse or beige-brown hair, fair, pink-toned skin, blue or grey eyes

Cue your hue: White and champagne blondes, mocha and chocolate browns

If you have: Golden or mid-brown hair, honey or olive-toned skin, green/brown eyes
Cue your hue: Rich nutty brown, claret red

If you have: Dark brown, mahogany hair, sallow skin, blue/grey eyes
Cue your hue: Plum and burgundy reds

If you have: Red hair, pale freckled skin, blue/grey eyes
Cue your hue: Auburn, gold and nutty browns

TLC FOR COLOUR

A colour change will alter the structure of your hair, so the way in which you treat it is crucial. Seek out products formulated specifically for coloured hair as run-of-the-mill shampoos can be too harsh and strip the colour, causing premature colour fade.

> 'You would not buy a cashmere sweater and wash it in harsh solution, so care for your coloured hair in the same gentle way.'
>
> **Jo Hansford**

The hair necessities of life

When it comes to hair, everybody's got a gripe, even celebrities. Too fine, too thick, too dull. Even those with seemingly perfect hair can have a wear-a-hat day. We've all seen hair gurus scurry around salons, wielding chrome-finished appliances and mysterious products. But there is a method to their madness: they only use what works.

BRUSH STROKES
A Cushion Brush
Use this for every hair type. A Mason and Pearson brush is universally accepted as *the* cushion brush as it's traditionally used to cleanse and add shine, plus give body to straight hair, along with detangling and smoothing out curly hair.

A Vent or Volumising Brush

Use this for root pickup. Widely spaced pins and air vent cut down on damaging drying time and are essential for extra root lift, volume and bounce.

A Small Round Brush

The only brush that can give curl to poker-straight fringes, add movement and root lift to medium and short hair, style curls and flicks, tame ends on layered styles and control permed hair. Use it for grooming on the go.

A Large Round Brush

Use this for making long waves straight. It's also perfect for creating or controlling waves and curls on straight hair, and great for smoothing and straightening curly hair.

A Paddle Brush

This brings polish to your hair – it glides through straight hair adding sleekness and shine. It's ideal for detangling and styling curly hair too, as the pins are widely spaced to prevent snagging or pulling.

'Using the right brush will massage the scalp and stimulate circulation, increasing the supply of nutrients to each hair. This helps promote healthy, strong hair growth.'

Trevor Sorbie

CLUED UP ABOUT COMBS

For taking out knots, use a wide-toothed comb: Hair is most fragile when it's wet. This comb affords great control.

For anti-static, use a wooden comb: Wood doesn't create friction like plastic can.

For teasing, lifting, pulling or tucking, use a tail comb: If you do any of the above to your hair this is a must-have.

For curl care, use a wide-toothed comb: Extremely gentle, which is key for TLC for long spirals.

> ★ **STAR BOX** *To increase volume in hair, brush against the growth pattern. A good way to do this is to tip the hair forwards and stroke from the nape to the ends.*

ESSENTIAL HAIR GOO AND WHAT THEY DO

Many a celebrity hairstylist avoids styling stress with their glittering clientèle by intrinsically knowing when the perfect product should come into play, how it works and, most importantly, how to handle it for best results. Hair magic that's worked on some of the world's most coveted manes can be yours too – straight from the shelf. It's just a case of being in the hair know.

Curl Boosters

A cross between a gel and a nourishing conditioner, a curl booster defines and enlivens natural curls and creates a soft, touchable texture. Separate washed hair into sections and work the product through from root to tip with your fingers, twisting as you go. Leave the hair to dry naturally.

Gels

Indispensable for slicking hair back into a sleek ponytail, also useful for getting to grips with an up-do, gels help glue hair into place. Similar to hairspray, they contain a large amount of polymer resins that dry into a firm hold and set your style into position. Rub gel between your palms, lightly run your hands over your hair and then comb through.

Glossers and Shiners

Excellent for giving an enviable glossy sheen to curly hair prone to flyaway ends and straight hair that lacks lustre, all glossers and shiners boost up the shine factor by coating the hair shaft with silicone. Rub the serum between your fingers and smooth it over your hair's surface. Or simply spritz with a shine spray.

Hairsprays or Fixing Sprays

Just the spray required for fixing a style into camera-ready position. Hold the nozzle six to 12 inches away from your head. The finer the hair, the further away you should hold the spray. Essential for creating root lift and spiking short hair.

Moulders and Shapers

Midway between a gel and a wax, they're a one-stop wonder for short hair. Use them on short hair that requires texturising and curly hair that craves definition. Apply them on dry hair and create twists and spikes to give all-over texture definition. Activate them by rubbing a small amount between your palms, then tease and ruffle your hair with your fingertips.

★ **STAR BOX** *Avoid mussed-up hair in the morning by laying your head on a satin pillowcase. 'Satin fabric allows your hair to gently slide cross it, as opposed to cotton, which causes more friction and disrupts the hair follicles,' says Charles Worthington.*

Mousses

Great for all hair types, mousses contain humectants that attract moisture to the hair shaft. They encourage body and definition to curly hair or enhance waves, thickness and volume in other types of hair. Spray a ball of mousse into your palms and spread it throughout wet hair. Scrunch the hair in your palms for maximum body and curl.

Straightening Balms

For any style that hates being kinky, these clever balms coat the hair shaft and smooth down the cuticle, making hair straighter. The risk of frizz is also reduced and protection is offered against heat-styling damage for a smooth-as-glass finish. If your hair is especially fine, opt for a lighter cream texture – thicker hair demands a heavier balm. Apply evenly on wet hair before blow-drying.

Volumisers

For limp hair that needs to look perkier and for wavy hair that needs lift and body, these deliver the va va voom factor. Now for the science bit: liquid resins double the width of the hair shaft by coating or fluffing out the cuticles. Apply volumisers by spraying or smoothing over wet hair before drying or styling. Massage them into the roots with your fingertips.

Waxes and Pomades

Brilliant for medium, thick and Afro hair to tame frizz or to define layers in shorter hairstyles. Rub a small amount between your palms then smooth sparingly onto dry hair. Separate out strands as you go to create oodles of texture.

EXTRA TOOLS OF THE TRADE

Professional Straightening Irons: These do an incredible job in turning an average hairdo into something altogether more glamorous. The results can be so impressive it's easy to get addicted to them. But use them sparingly, as you are literally ironing out the moisture from your hair.

A Super-powerful Hairdryer: Power can be everything when drying hair. Look for both hot and cold settings. The hot hair dries and the cold shot helps to lock in your style.

Hair Bungees: Elastic bands can tear and rip the hair. Bungees are great for securing hair in a ponytail without damaging the cuticles.

Curling Irons: Crucial for adding glamour waves and creating super curls. But like the straightening irons, don't overuse them unless you want straw-like texture to your hair.

Extra-large Velcro Rollers: If you have to throw a look together in 20 minutes, these are an unbelievably fast fix. Wrap the entire head around five rollers, do your make-up, remove the rollers and hair presto, hair to rival that of any Tinseltown starlet!

20 INSIDER TAKEAWAY SALON SECRETS

Celebrity stylists seem to wave magic hands over hair, getting it to fall perfectly, look lustrous and hold its shape, while when we try, it often flops. What are the style secrets to achieving hair worthy of the red-carpet treatment at home?

Here leading celebrity hair gurus reveal some of their tricks of the trade along with take-home tips that can really help your hair look as though it belongs on the silver screen.

1. One key reason hair comes away from the salon looking indecently shiny is that in a salon hair is never washed in the bath. Specially designed salon basins let hair flow freely in one direction under clean water. When washing hair at home, hop in the shower or bend over the edge of a bath and use a shower attachment to get your hair really clean.

2. Using masses of shampoo isn't the route to cleaner hair. Instead, it's down to methodical application and proper massage. Spread a dessertspoonful of shampoo between your hands, lift your hair at the scalp and distribute the shampoo as evenly as possible. Then, concentrating on a small section of your scalp at a time, massage your scalp, using the pads of

your fingertips in a circular motion. This not only helps dislodge grime, it also contributes to healthier-looking hair by boosting circulation.

3. An awful lot of towels are used at the salon, but it's all for a good reason: it speeds drying time with minimum trauma to your hair. Follow suit at home by first blotting – not scrubbing – wet hair with a fluffy towel to get rid of excess moisture, then wrapping it in another dry towel for a further few minutes. The more your hair is allowed to dry naturally, the less time you waste on heat styling and hair abuse.

4. Rinse, rinse, rinse. 'Insufficient rinsing, especially along the hairline, can result in residue that dulls the hair,' says celebrity hairdresser Richard Ward. 'Leading trichologists [hair doctors] agree we should rinse for at least two minutes to remove residue. You also need plenty of water, not only to wash away the grease and dirt lifted by the shampoo, but also to activate the conditioning agents in your haircare products.'

5. If you don't arm yourself with a decent dryer, you're wasting your time. You need one with at least 1,500 watts of power and a variety of heat and speed settings for ultimate flexibility. And don't even think about picking up your dryer until your hair is 80 per cent dry. No amount of heat styling is going to make any impact on wet hair – all you're doing is knocking the body out of it. Try a final rinse in mineral water – a tactic rumoured to be used by Jennifer Lopez to flatten the cuticles and boost the shine factor.

6. 'When there's no time to wash your hair, revive your

hairstyle with a blow-drying spray,' advocates Charles Worthington. 'To add volume, spritz it directly onto the roots then blow-dry, paying particular attention to the root area.'

7. Charles Worthington also divulges, 'When coming into a hot, steamy atmosphere like a party from the cold night air, backcomb your hair at the roots. This will instantly keep the hair big all night and make it better able to cope with the change in temperature.'

8. Many hair problems, from brittleness to lack of shine, can be attributed to nutritional deficiencies. Poor hair growth or loss of colour can be a sign of zinc deficiency. So boost up on your supplement quota or look to natural sources such as oysters, Brazil nuts and steak. When Jennifer Aniston chopped her hair off, she regretted it. She tempted back Rapunzel-like tresses by supplementing her diet with silicon.

9. If hair is fragile or weak, it has probably been fried and distressed as a result of over-processing. When celebrity hair is constantly being styled for photo shoots and prepped for film roles, the damage can be so severe the hair can start to resemble candyfloss. To the rescue: a protein-based intensive conditioning treatment to help retain moisture and repair the hair's keratin.

10. To add volume to limp locks, start in the shower. Shampoo with a volumising product, then apply light conditioner to the ends only. When your hair is 60 per cent dry, apply a body-boosting spray to the roots.

Blow-dry by lifting sections of your hair with your fingers and aiming the heat at your roots.

11. Don't dry against the direction of hair growth. Angle the nozzle towards the ends for super smoothness.

12. 'Nicole Kidman likes me to straighten her hair when she's pulling out all the glamour stops,' says her stylist Kerry Warn. 'I usually blow-dry her hair straight, them smooth out the texture with straightening irons to give a modern and sexy feel. Don't try to blow-dry curls straight unless you've got 45 minutes to an hour spare. It's a disaster when people do the front and haven't got time for the back.'

13. To disguise dark roots between salon colour touch-ups, zigzag your parting by flipping the hair over to the left and then to the right. It camouflages the re-growth line. Or use a few strokes of brown or black mascara, depending on your hair colour, to put greys into hiding. Wash it out at night.

14. Work with your hair texture as much as possible, not against it. And keep styling products to the minimum – three at the max. Stake out the right ones for your hair and then try them out.

15. Be sparing with silicone-based products – they can weigh the hair down, ultimately making it look life-less and delivering a 'fake' plastic-looking shine instead of a natural-looking one.

16. Switch the hand with which you hold the dryer when working on different sides of the head. It feels odd at first, but it makes for a more symmetrical result.

17. Attach the correct styling nozzle to the dryer. It's

amazing how many people don't bother and then wonder why their hair looks a flop. It's essential to have a diffuser to define and control curls and a metal nozzle to direct air flow for straighter styles.

18. Get used to finishing your look by styling with your fingers. If you watch top stylists, especially those on photo sessions, they play with the hair until it starts to fall into shape. Dragging brushes through a near-finished style can ruin the shape.

19. If you have ultra-fine hair, avoid applying a finishing spray on top of your style as it will be too heavy and remove fullness and bounce. An alternative is to bend your head down and apply spray to the under layers for lift without heaviness.

20. Don't be afraid to backcomb. It can transform a style. The key to not harming your hair is to tease volume into it with a comb and later tease it out again using a big, soft brush.

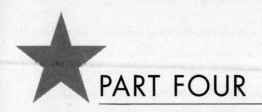

PART FOUR

The skinny on dropping weight

Once upon a time stars were celebrated for their full and generous figures: think Marilyn Monroe and Jayne Mansfield. But that's where the fairy story ends. Today, there's no question about it: Hollywood likes its women thin, and for some stars, dieting has almost become a competitive sport. If they can't make the headlines because of their work, why not because of their new figure?

In the past the word 'diet' had a certain connotation of shame – it meant you were losing your grip – but today every A-lister worth her low-sodium salt has a nutritionist and a personal chef on her payroll and talks non-stop about some kind of diet she lives by. American style bible *W* has even been quoted as saying 'Diets are the new religion.' Far from feeling inhibited about talking weight, stars openly discuss their eating habits. Having some kind of diet on the go is *de rigueur*. Gwyneth Paltrow and Madonna have had a bonding experience over their strict macrobiotic diet of brown rice and green lentils and Jennifer Aniston – she of the high-protein body – successfully dropped around two stone and reportedly turned the cast of *Friends* onto her Zone programme. 'I hate it when self-worth is measured by how much you weigh,' she says. But nonetheless she gave up snacks, along with butter and mayonnaise. Many of these famously endorsed diets then become stop-the-press news in themselves. In essence, A-listers have glamorised the practice of taking off weight.

> '**Celebrities need to look their best. It's their job and their physical image takes a leading role in how effective and how successful they are at being a celebrity.**'
>
> **David Marshall aka The BodyDoctor,** *personal trainer to Rachel Weisz and Sophie Dahl*

Whether we like to swallow it or not, some stars are just born lucky.

> '**I'm blessed with a quick metabolism, so I can eat more or less what I like.**'
>
> **Cameron Diaz**

But the blueprint of success for many a celebrity is sheer naked ambition and hard work. And that's never truer than when they're sweating into shape. They know the camera easily adds on 10lb (4.5kg) and packing on the pounds could mean packing their bags when it comes to talking major film roles.

When it comes to losing weight, nothing is too tough or too bizarre. And nothing can be more confusing. What one expert says to eat, the other says not. The upshot is to literally digest the following advice and choose an eating plan that suits you and your lifestyle without feeling that you're depriving yourself. In truth there's no great secret to losing weight: you simply eat less and move more and make it your way of life. Celebrities don't really know any more than we do. They simply hire people to tell them what to eat and when. And that's what this section offers: the best guidance from those who advise the tightest butts in town!

The diets on A-listers' lips

Catherine Zeta Jones followed the Zone diet to get into shape for her nuptials to Michael Douglas, and Elizabeth Hurley is reported to let her blood group dictate what she eats. You've no doubt read about the diets the stars follow to guarantee they look lean for all those big-carpet moments. But what do they actually involve? Here's the low-down.

The Atkins Diet

The Atkins Diet is nothing new; it's been around since the seventies. Its low-carbohydrate high-protein basis can result in quick weight loss and because of this it has gained a huge celebrity fan base including Jennifer Lopez and Minnie Driver. Devotees have reported losing between 10 and 30lb (4.5 and 13.5kg) a month.

Developed by the late Dr Robert Atkins, the diet advocates limiting carbohydrate intake. The philosophy is that the body metabolises carbohydrates first. Cut down on carbs and you will burn fat. So you can eat all the protein and fat you want and bring about quick weight loss. Hence the Atkins Diet appeals to any member of the celebrity fraternity looking for a fast way to slim down into a designer dress. Meat, cheese and eggs are all on the menu. Fruit, bread, grains and potatoes are not. It's worth bearing in mind, though, that this kind of high-protein, low-carb diet goes against most public health professionals' advice.

The Blood Group Diet

As far as diets go, this is as personal as it gets. Naturopath Dr Peter D'Adamo, author of *Eat Right for Your Type*, has taken Hollywood by storm. He believes that your blood group type is the blueprint to how you burn your calories, which foods you should eat and how you benefit from certain types of exercise. But how does finding out your blood group guarantee to melt away the pounds? D'Adamo believes that a chemical reaction occurs between your blood and foods as they are digested. Lectins (diverse and abundant proteins found in food) may be incompatible with your blood group and adverse side-effects may occur, such as putting on weight, feeling sluggish or finding it difficult to handle stress or illness.

Why so many celebrities have opted for this way of eating is because it's tailor-made for their own personal DNA. They have been convinced that a diet shaped to their individual blood type works because you are able to follow a clear, logical, scientifically researched plan based on your cellular profile. For instance, blood group O is classed as the Hunter and benefits from eating meat, fish, vegetables and fruit. Foods to avoid are wheat, corn, lentils, cabbage and cauliflower.

The Zone

This is a diet that is said to have you burning fat 24 hours a day. Take inspiration from Jennifer Aniston and Sarah Michelle Gellar, who have both been put into the 'Zone' and have their diet delivered on set. Developed by Dr Barry Sears, whose recommendations are based on 15 years of research as a bio-nutritionist, the Zone diet meals are made up of 40 per cent carbohydrate, 30 per cent protein and 30 per cent fat. Dr Sears concludes that combining food properly and regulating insulin levels help the body burn old fat instead of producing new fat. And by eating the proper ratio of carbs to fat to protein, you can begin controlling your insulin production. This eating plan suggests you graze during the day on six small meals rather than three main ones to keep insulin levels consistent. Approved dishes include lots of chicken, fish and even bacon, sausages and eggs. But with limited amounts of carbohydrates.

The Macrobiotic Diet

Gwyneth Paltrow and Madonna attribute their well-being to eating macrobiotically. This diet is based on principles and practices that have been known to philosophers and physicians throughout history. It comes from the Greek: *macro* means 'long' and *bios* means 'life'. Mainly a vegan eating plan, it focuses on eating more wholegrains, beans, vegetables and fruit that benefit both personal health and the health of the environment. Meat, animal fats, eggs, poultry and dairy products are off the agenda. Both the aforementioned A-listers attribute their energies and slim figures to eating 'clean foods' that come straight from the earth, and eating regularly and less. Madonna is said to like seaweed soup and drinks such as roasted bancha twig tea. Proper chewing – around 50 times per mouthful – and not eating two to three hours before sleeping are also in the macrobiotic lifestyle rulebook if you fancy shaping up like these two health-conscious stars.

The LifeFood Diet

The antithesis of Atkins: a low-fat diet that comprises fruit, vegetables, wholegrains, beans, sushi and soy products in their natural forms. Fashion designer Donna Karan is looking sexier than ever before and has dropped 20lb (9kg) in a year thanks to this diet. Claiming to feel 'nurtured' by it, she has it cooked up by her own personal chef, who serves such delicacies as coconut cucumber soup. In this eating plan cooking food is mainly frowned upon, but if you do, nothing should be heated to more than 108°C to keep essential nutrients intact. The usual suspects – anything processed, refined, canned or genetically engineered – are seriously off the menu.

The Food Combination Diet

This is otherwise known as the Hay Diet, as it was Dr William Hay who developed it over 80 years ago. It is based on the principle that carbohydrates, or starches, require a mainly alkaline medium to be digested properly, while protein requires an acid medium. So, put simply, the idea is to avoid eating starches and protein at the same meal for more balanced and efficient digestion. The pulling power for this diet is that it allows you to eat anything you like as long as it's properly combined. Theoretically, a big plate of fries is allowed as long as you don't eat fish with it. The downside? It can be time-consuming to work out all the right combinations! But hey, that's where personal chefs earn their money!

The Carbohydrates Addict Diet

This diet was developed by husband-and-wife combo Drs Rachael and Richard Heller, who were both overweight and initially devised this diet for themselves. They now have a bestselling book under their much smaller belts and a thriving clinic in America that treats hundreds of people each week. The diet promises impressive weight loss by simply replacing refined sugar, pasta, potatoes and bread with everything else, such as fat, meat, non-starchy vege-tables and dairy products.

Courteney Cox, a fan of this eating plan, says, 'If I eat pasta for dinner, I gain weight. If I eat protein, I lose weight.' According to the authors, carbohydrate addiction is caused by a hormonal imbalance – an over-release of the hormone insulin that is brought on when carbohydrate foods are eaten. Among its many jobs, insulin signals the body to take in food and then signals it to store the food energy in the form of fat. The Hellers' theory is that because carbohydrates turn into sugar, which in turn creates insulin, they cause excessive weight gain.

The Sugar Busters! Diet

Sugar is seen as pure white, deliciously sweet and nutritionally vacant by many nutritionists. And there's little doubt that it makes you fat. So three doctors and a scientist came out with a diet called Sugar Busters! and it's the slim-down strategy for many a star. According to the authors, this is a nutritional lifestyle, not just another fad diet. It is about how, what and when to eat. Begin by cutting sugar – and this doesn't mean just the refined processed sugar found in biscuits, cakes and starchy foods like bread, but also the unrefined and unprocessed sugar or carbohydrates found in some fruit and vegetables like bananas, raisin, carrots and potatoes. Confused? The key to this diet is to avoid foods that have what's called a high glycaemic index. The glycaemic index measures how high blood sugar rises after you eat. Many carbohydrates score highly, since they are broken down in the body into sugar. This drives up production of the hormone insulin. According to the authors, when there is too much insulin, the body stores excess sugar as fat.

The Weil Diet

Physician and alternative medicine man Dr Andrew Weil defends the good old healthfood diet: low in saturated fats, low in protein and high in fresh fruit, vegetables and wholegrains. He advises 50–60 per cent carbohydrates, 30 per cent fats and 10–20 per cent protein. He repeatedly criticises the Zone diet, warning that the nitrogen released by all of that protein potentially damages the liver and kidneys. Dr Weil believes that we would have better diets if we got away from the idea that meat should be the centrepiece of a meal and we ate more fish like salmon. The bottom line of his nutritional recommendations is: do not eat partially hydrogenated fats such as hard margarine and processed foods such as pastries. Do consume large quantities of omega-3 fats, mostly low glycaemic index carbohydrates and only small amounts of foods that contain flour or sugar. *Friends* star Lisa Kudrow claims that through following this diet she has learned the difference between cravings, physical hunger and body satisfaction.

Ways to Spot a Fad Diet

★ It only has one ingredient in the name. Living solely on cabbage, grapefruit or eggs will only work in the short term, as your calorie intake will drop to semi-starvation level. Plus there's only so much cabbage a girl can take unless she wants to be a social outcast!

★ You need to be armed with a chemistry degree to work out different food combinations that you are allowed to eat. Just remember, your body was designed to multitask!

★ It boasts you'll keep the weight off forever. Yeah, if you stick to eating nothing! Anytime you come off a calorie-controlled diet you risk putting back on the pounds. The only fail-safe way to keep the weight off is by sensible eating and exercise.

★ Foods your mum always encouraged you to stock up on are now all of a sudden the Devil's food!

Can bananas really store excess sugar as fat? Perhaps it's all taking the science of nutrition a little too literally.

★ It claims weight loss is easy peasy. And bikini waxes are completely painless! Losing weight takes discipline and commitment – and it ain't that easy.

Eat smart, look the part

When British actress Samantha Morton was handed the script for her Hollywood role in *Minority Report* opposite Tom Cruise, she realised that she would be wearing a leather catsuit. That's when she decided to call upon the help of personal trainer Kathryn Freeland, who not only makes stars sweat by helping them to tone up for their parts but oversees their nutrition too.

> 'Dieting makes you fat and miserable. Fad diets do work, but only while you're on them. They give you a guide to eat less than your needs. You lose weight, but the weight loss is not permanent because you are not losing fat.'
>
> **Kathryn Freeland,** *personal trainer to Samantha Morton and Cate Blanchett*

For instance, on a high-protein/low-carbohydrate diet most of the weight loss in the beginning of the diet is water weight. So you see the number on the scales going down, but the upshot is you aren't losing fat. Once you break the diet, you gain the weight back immediately. According to Freeland, the only way to break the fad-diet cycle is to stop the lunacy of eating cabbage soup or whatever every day or depriving yourself of carbohydrates and start eating healthily.

Kathryn's Absolute Diet is given to all the celebrities who walk through her doors. She says: 'I give an eating plan that people can actually follow and not feel hungry. It's realistic and allows you to have a little bit of everything you want. Use your common sense about what to eat and when: alcohol and a curry before bedtime are not going to do your waistline any favours. Arm yourself with a little knowledge and just concentrate on getting it right every day. Before you know it, you won't even have to think about it.'

A typical day on the Absolute Diet would look something like this:

Breakfast:	Fruit and natural yoghurt
Snack:	Walnuts or pumpkin seeds
Lunch:	Tuna or chicken sandwich with brown bread
Snack:	Cherries
Dinner:	Cous cous with roasted vegetables and feta cheese

The Absolute Nutrition Lifestyle Guide

★ Eat sensibly. A little of everything does you good.

★ Vary the types of food eaten as often as possible for maximum nutrient intake.

★ Snack within two to three hours of your last meal otherwise your body wastes muscle and stores fat, which slows down your metabolism.

★ Eat a small carbohydrate meal (pasta or rice) before your exercise session and a protein meal (meat or eggs) afterwards.

★ Leave two hours for a meal to digest before hitting the treadmill.

★ If you are feeling tired, look to a banana or small glucose drink instead of chocolate.

★ Eat five portions per day of vegetables, salad and fruit. A glass of diluted orange juice can count as one portion.

★ Eat fish four times per week.

★ Eat white meat two to three times per week.

★ Eat red meat one to two times per week.

★ Try to grill, steam or poach instead of roasting and frying.

★ Avoid adding salt to your meal.

'Never order a fruit salad as dessert. The different sugars from the different fruits combine and ferment in the stomach, causing it to bloat and distend.'

David Marshall aka The BodyDoctor

THE GREAT FRIDGE MAKEOVER

Every refrigerator tells a story. Stars knows this like nobody else, which is why they employ tough-talking personal eating trainers or diet coaches. Yes, they really do exist! Eating trainers whip A-list butts into shape by striding into their luxurious homes and rifling through their food cupboards and fridges, ditching the bad food. They even talk stars through restaurant menus and retrain their eating habits – for a price, of course.

Nancy Kennedy is one of the most sought-after nutrition experts in California. Julia Roberts and Lara Flynn Boyle have both benefited from her advice. Her aim is to make her clients become healthy and strong in mind as well as body, and she firmly believes in moderation. 'The size of your portions is very important,' she states. 'A piece of chicken or fish should fit into the palm of your hand. No bigger. Ever.' Her foodie hate is processed food. 'It's total trash and drives me crazy,' she says. 'Whole dairy products, processed deli meats and all white stuff – sugar, white flour and white pasta – should all be thrown out. Proteins are lean and firm and will do the same for your body. Likewise for bad carbohydrates that are soft and puffy.'

Other nutrition tips from Kennedy include thinking ahead. 'Keep a protein bar – low fat, low sugar and low carb – in your bag, so if you feel peckish you won't feel tempted to buy a bar of chocolate. Think ahead and stock up at the market so you're never caught without good food in your fridge and when travelling take your own food for the plane ride.'

Jackie Keller is another food expert. An LA-based

dietician and teacher who heads up and runs Nutrifit, a gourmet-food delivery service providing mouthwatering and nutritionally sound meals, she's catered for Lucy Liu, Uma Thurman and Daryl Hannah. Keller's menus are customised to individual nutritional needs and taste preference. A one-day sample menu may consist of: German apple pancakes for breakfast, a wild berry fruit smoothie for a mid-morning snack, pan-seared chicken with curry and chutney for lunch, hummus with baked pitta chips for an afternoon snack and roasted tomato soup, rosemary-scented lamb with cous cous and Mediterranean vegetables for dinner.

Uma Thurman's Favourite Wild Berry Smoothie

½ cup of mixed frozen unsweetened berries including blueberries, strawberries and raspberries
1 cup of unsweetened apple juice
3oz (75g) tofu
½ small banana
Blend until completely smooth. Drink and enjoy!

Jackie reveals: 'Uma Thurman is an adventurous cook and so an adventurous eater. She likes vegetarian dishes made with tofu and Asian-style food. Although, like many stars, she's concerned about eating too many carbohydrates, I include favourable carbs like wholegrains with tons of vegetables, along with lean poultry and fish.'

This kind of diet worked a treat for Uma when she had to drop 25lb (11kg) post baby for her role in Quentin Tarantino's film *Kill Bill*.

Jackie Keller's Happy Eater Tips

★ Eat fruit instead of sugar. Think of a mouthwatering piece of fruit as your sugar. Take the ripest, therefore sweetest, piece of fruit and eat it at room temperature. That way it has more flavour.

★ Uma Thurman has a very sweet tooth and one that tempts is my sugar-free fruit cobblers. I combine two of each type of stone fruit such as peaches, nectarines, plums and apricots coarsely chopped, then add a sprinkling of walnuts and oatmeal for texture – crunchy food is very satisfying – then a spoonful of frozen apple juice concentrate and a tiny bit of canola oil. When these are all baked together, the sugars caramelise and the taste explodes.

★ For foods loaded with calories, such as nuts, cheese and chocolate, chop, grate or shave them so they go further and then put them on the top or outside of the food. The theory is, if you stir them in, your eye won't spy them, so your brain won't realise you've had them.

★ Think of food as your friend, not your enemy. Eating sensibly will help you lose weight; starving or avoiding meals will cause your body to hold onto its reserves and actually thwart your weight-loss efforts.

★ Don't be ruled by the scales. Aim for a happy weight. That's where you've got your body and mind together. Aim to take enough exercise so you start feeling good enough about yourself so you don't have to comfort eat.

★ Take time out to prepare fresh food for yourself. Lots

of takeaways and pre-prepared food will drain your vitality and add on the pounds.

READY, STEADY, GO . . .

If you're not on an A-list salary you may as well forget enlisting the skills of a diet coach. But opening a woman's fridge is much like looking into her medicine cabinet: a quick scan can reveal a great deal about her life.

'The bottom line is that most people know what to eat but don't have the discipline to follow it through,' remarks Kathryn Freeland. 'The key is making subtle changes.'

To get you on the right track, why not follow the Traffic Lite Diet foundation of better eating? A simple, easy-to-follow programme, it is in line with many top nutritionists' thinking.

Green: Go Ahead

Cereals and Bread	High-fibre multi-grained bread, fortified breakfast cereals, cous cous, wholemeal pasta, oatmeal and rice
Meat and Alternatives	Broiled chicken (no skin), lean ham, tofu, turkey (no skin), very lean red meat
Dairy Foods	Cottage cheese, feta cheese, low-fat soft cheese, low-fat yoghurt, skimmed milk, non-fat sour cream
Fish	Shellfish, whitefish – broiled, steamed or baked
Flavoured Olive Oils	Non-stick cooking sprays

Fruit and Vegetables	All fruit – apples, pears, oranges – and vegetables, fresh and frozen. Beans (canned and dried), baked potatoes and boiled potatoes
Sweets	Dark chocolate with 70 per cent cocoa solids. Just a couple of squares can be more satisfying than cheaper milkier chocolate that contains more sugar, fat and butter.
Drinks and Soups	Clear soups, limited coffee, lots of water, fresh fruit juices, diet sodas
Others	Herbs, mustard, spices, vinegar, Worcestershire sauce

Yellow: Don't Overdo It

Cereals and Bread	Crunchy cereals, granola cereals
Meat	Lean cuts of beef, lean cuts of pork, lean cuts of lamb, lean bacon, liver
Dairy Foods	Poached eggs, boiled eggs, cheddar, Parmesan, Brie, Edam
Fish	Trout, herring, salmon
Fats and Oils	Vegetable oils, sunflower, olive oil – a little for cooking – low-fat spreads
Fruit and Vegetables	Go easy on mashed potatoes. Add only 2 per cent milk or non-fat sour cream.

Nuts	Most. Eat only a few at a time.
Sweets	Honey, marmalade, jam, peanut butter
Biscuits and Desserts	Low-fat ice cream, cakes and cereal bars
Drinks and Soups	Low-fat hot cocoa, unsweetened cappuccino, low-fat soups
Others	Low-fat mayonnaise, non-fat dressings, thin-crust vegetable pizza

Red: Stop and Think!

Cereals and Bread	Croissants, frosted cereals loaded with sugar
Meat	Bacon, salami, sausages, hamburgers, visible fat on meat
Dairy Foods	Full-fat cheese, coffee creamers, condensed milk, cream, cream cheese, fried eggs, whole milk, full-fat yoghurt
Fish	Fried fish and fish spreads
Fats and Oils	Butter
Fruit and Vegetables	Avocado, canned fruit in syrup, chips, roasted potatoes
Nuts	Salted nuts

Sweets	Chocolate, chocolate spread, fudge and toffees
Biscuits and Desserts	Cheesecakes, dairy ice cream, pudding, most ready-made cakes, biscuits, pastry
Alcoholic and Cream-based Drinks	Full-fat milkshakes. For alcohol, stick to two units a day – that's two small glasses of wine or two shots of spirits.
Others	Creamy and oily dressings, mayonnaise, meat-based pizzas or extra-cheese pizzas, savoury sauces made with fat or cream, fast-food meals

Drop the weight you want

The road to weight-loss success begins with choosing the right plan. Whether your aim is to drop a little weight or a couple of dress sizes, the basic principles are the same: consume fewer calories than you burn off. However, someone who wants to drop 5lb (2.5kg) faces different challenges from someone who wants to lose 30lb (13.5kg). To avoid failure and guarantee success, you need to tailor your weight-loss scheme to your personal goal. This is advice that has been shared with me by numerous nutrition experts over the years. Follow it and you've got nothing to lose but your weight!

YOU WANT TO DITCH 5LB (2.5KG)

★ Cut back on sugar and refined starches and hold back on the alcohol. Keep a food diary: note what you eat for the next week then scan it for hidden sources of unnecessary and nutrient-free calories. By eliminating 250 calories a day – that's just two glasses of wine – you can lose half a pound a week quite easily.

★ Drink like a fish. I'm talking water, not spirits! Those 5lb could be fluid that your body is happily holding onto in response to hormone fluctuations.

★ While tweaking your diet is more than half the battle, the right exercise regime can help too. Vary your routine. Remember muscles have memory and can quickly become bored. Muscle burns more calories than fat, so add strength training into your cardiovascular workout.

★ **STAR BOX** *Start the day with a pink organic grapefruit. The bioflavonoids found in the pith and skin segments are anti-inflammatory agents, making it great for the digestive system.*

YOU WANT TO DITCH 15LB (6.5KG)

★ Skip the takeout lunches and delivery pizzas. These are all foods with an unknown calorie count. Rustle up your own recipes and you'll have a better idea of how many calories you're consuming.

★ Eat more fruit and vegetables. These are high in fibre, so they'll fill you up but with fewer calories.

★ Pinpoint when you comfort eat. Most people indulge at the same time every day, usually between lunch and dinner or dinner and bedtime. If you're guilty, do something else that occupies your mind rather than snacking.

YOU WANT TO DITCH 30LB (13.5KG)

★ Seek the advice of a professional. To lose this amount, you'll need to make major lifestyle changes. An expert, whether a doctor, dietician or weight management expert, can help you make changes safely and effectively.

★ Say nice things to yourself instead of giving yourself a hard time. Affirmations are great, but say them with conviction. 'I am getting nearer to the person I want to be every day' is a great one.

★ Make one small change every day. Start by modifying your breakfast one week, your lunch the next. That way, you'll have less to adjust to. Tell yourself you have an amazing body – you do – and really look after it instead of neglecting it and filling it with junk.

★ Get enough shuteye. Not sleeping enough can hinder your chances of dropping weight. When you're sleep-deprived, your body produces higher levels of a stress hormone called cortisol, which keeps you alert and causes sugar cravings.

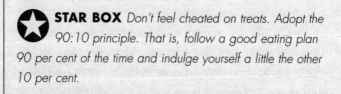

STAR BOX *Don't feel cheated on treats. Adopt the 90:10 principle. That is, follow a good eating plan 90 per cent of the time and indulge yourself a little the other 10 per cent.*

Spice up your tastebuds!

Gayle Reichler, nutritionist at the star-studded Avon Salon & Spa in New York, reckons the best way to 'lighten up' is to intensify your food's flavour while losing some fat and calories. Here are some of her secrets on rustling up and revving up healthy low-calorie food.

Salsa and dip: 'Whether sweet or savoury, there's no better way than marinating meat, chicken or fish in salsa to add a healthy shot of vitamins and jazz up your meal,' Reichler says. Concoct your own version by blending either tomatoes or soft fruit such as peaches or mangoes with red onion, wine vinegar and a dash of olive oil.

Shake things up: Gayle explains that shakes and smoothies are perfect for supplying healthy doses of calcium, particularly if you start with skimmed milk or low-fat yoghurt. 'To add fibre and vitamins without unnecessary calories, use fresh fruit instead of juice,' she reveals.

Think green: 'Vegetables are very low in calories and high in nutritional value, plus they add fibre, flavour and crunch to any meal,' Gayle says. Add chopped carrots, red pepper and even fresh peas to chicken and tuna salads or layer sandwiches with tomatoes, sprouts, cucumber and watercress.

Mix and match: Salads don't have to be limited to vegetables. 'Adding fruit will make for a much more interesting and fulfilling meal,' Gayle reveals. 'Apples, peaches, pears and apricots are wonderful complements to meats and light cheeses.'

FOOD FOR HIGH-VOLTAGE ENERGY

If there's one thing celebrities can't have a short supply of, it's energy. How do they get it?

The Joshi Clinic is London's foremost complementary health centre and is one of the celebrities' best-kept secrets. Founder and practitioner of the clinic is Dr Nish Joshi, who treats the likes of Cate Blanchett, Sadie Frost, Jude Law, Kate Moss and Ralph Fiennes. He explains, 'Most problems stem from past deeds: too much drink, lack of exercise, misuse of drugs – recreational and antibiotics – generally bad living habits. But I don't dwell in the past, I undo the past and propel patients into the future.'

When it comes to nutritional and dietary support, Dr Joshi gives patients clear and concise guidance on balanced dietary needs for a healthy, energised body.

'Your body needs more than just calories to keep going. Nutrients like fibre, vitamins, minerals and essential fats help provide energy over the course of the day.'

Dr Nish Joshi, *Complementary therapist to Jude Law, Kate Moss and Sadie Frost*

Dr Joshi advocates dividing your plate into imaginary thirds and filling each third with one of the following nutrient-rich foods:

1. Wholegrains: brown rice, oats and wholewheat bread
2. Colourful fruit and vegetables: berries, cantaloupe, leafy greens and red peppers
3. Proteins: chicken, cottage cheese, eggs, tofu, tuna

To make sure you don't overeat, which can cause drowsiness, he recommends using an 8-inch (20cm) plate or limiting your grain portion to the size of a balled fist and your protein portion to that of a deck of cards. Then add some healthy fats by drizzling about a tablespoon of flaxseed oil or olive oil onto your food. 'The fibre in grains, fruits and vegetables helps ensure a steady supply of energy,' he says, 'because it slows your body's absorption of carbohydrates, a key energy source. Colourful fruits and vegetables provide energy-producing vitamins and minerals, and lean protein and healthy fats satisfy you so you're not weak with hunger. Omega-3 fats, found in flaxseed oil and fatty fish, help to keep your brain humming. All these foods work synergistically together to keep your body on full alert.'

'If you're trying to lose weight, it's best to avoid carbohydrates after 4 p.m. Your metabolism starts to slow down after that time and is more likely to store the calories.'

Dr Nish Joshi

★ **STAR BOX** *Try and cut out sugar as much as possible, especially hidden sugar in processed foods. Sugar kills, fat doesn't. Eat oily fish, grilled chicken with green vegetables and green salads of raw spinach and asparagus tips.*

THE PARTY GIRL'S NUTRITION BOOSTERS

Being a star doesn't allow you to be a party pooper. Looking like a celebrity means being ready to face the camera anytime. And food plays an enormous part in this – more so than the best concealer. As that old chestnut goes, true beauty is inner beauty – and although you may scoff, it's true. Feed yourself with large plates of pasta or Chinese takeaways every day and watch what happens to your skin.

'Just as the wrong foods can age you – right before your eyes – the right foods can take away years. Once you see and feel the results that the right foods can deliver, you will realise that there is a facelift in your fridge.'

Nicholas Perricone, *dermatologist to Julia Roberts and Kim Cattrall*

In the time it took you to read this small paragraph, you could be dramatically improving the nutritional quality of your diet – celebrity style. Sounds hard to believe, but it's a fact. Here are the super foods that nutritionists personally recommend. You'll find that many personal chefs will always have them on their grocery list to keep their well-nourished stars literally shining.

The Top 20 Superfoods: The Party Girl's Essential Nibbles

Apples: Unpeeled apples are rich in fibre that benefits digestion and lowers cholesterol by sweeping it out of your intestines. Because they contain fibre and fructose – a fruit sugar – apples have a low rating on the glycaemic index, which means they keep blood sugar levels steady and hunger at bay longer than other types of fruit.

Bell Peppers: Green, yellow and orange bell peppers are among the best vegetable sources of vitamin C, but red bell peppers are even better. They provide three times as much vitamin C as oranges.

Berries: They contain phytochemicals that prevent cell damage that may lead to cancer. One cup of raspberries supplies a third of your daily requirement of fibre.

Brazil Nuts: Dr Nish Joshi recommends taking two Brazil nuts a day, as you would a supplement. That serving provides roughly 150mcg of selenium – a powerful anti-oxidant and necessary for metabolism.

Broccoli: Green vegetables should find their way into a meal at least once a day. Chemicals in broccoli and other vegetables such as cauliflower and cabbage have been found to harbour a special anti-cancer chemical called sulfor-aphane that assists the body in detoxifying carcinogenic substances that enter it via the environment or diet.

Brown Rice: Provides a good dose of the bone-building minerals, magnesium and phosphorous as well as mood-enhancing B vitamins.

Cabbage: Lightly steamed or shredded raw cabbage is an excellent skin saver. If you can bear it, drink cabbage water. It makes for an excellent blood cleanser.

Eggs: Many women in Celebville, including Jennifer Lopez, are fans of egg-white omelettes. Eggs are among the most nutrient-rich foods, providing ¼ oz (6.25g) of the most complete, absorbable and usable protein as well as 13 essential nutrients for just 70 calories.

Grapefruit: Precious for its fibre, pectin and vitamin C content. The bioflavonoids found in the pith and skin segments are blood vessel strengtheners, anti-inflammatory agents, powerful antioxidants and fighters of infection.

Green Tea: Rich in polyphenols – strong chemicals that wage war against free radicals. Dr Joshi also reports there's new research suggesting that polyphenols may stimulate weight loss by boosting the metabolism.

Kiwi Fruit: Contains twice the vitamin C of an orange and four times the fibre of a stick of celery. Teeming with vitamin E and potassium. Great for juicing, or just cut in half and eat the flesh.

Lemons: Vital in the quest for healthier-looking skin. A great cleanser, packed with vitamin C (more than that of oranges) and bioflavonoids. Wake up to a glass of hot water with a slice of lemon.

Mangoes: The single best fruit source of cancer-fighting carotenoids. Also rich in the key antioxidant vitamins C and E.

Mushrooms: Asian mushrooms such as shiitake and maitake have traditionally been eaten to increase longevity. Studies suggest that compounds in these have anti-cancer, anti-viral and immune-boosting effects.

Papaya: Teeming with beta carotene and vitamin C, this tropical fruit is an immune-system booster and cancer fighter as well as being a valuable source of soluble fibre which helps lower cholesterol.

Salmon: A personal favourite of Dr Nicholas Perricone. He believes that the flesh of salmon is the ultimate de-wrinkling food because of its anti-inflammatory qualities and its very high levels of the skin-tightening chemical dimethylaminoethanol (DMAE). 'It's your magic bullet for great skin tone, keeping your face firm and contoured,' he divulges.

Sea Vegetables: Kelp and kale are regulars with the stars as a fresh vegetable food. Seaweed from non-toxic waters is a source of valuable minerals, including calcium, chromium, cobalt, iron, iodine, manganese and zinc.

Sprouted Seeds, Beans and Grains: One of the most nurturing and nourishing food groups. Plus they're great for the skin. Sprouting mung beans, pumpkin seeds, lentils chick peas and aduki beans provide an abundant source of nourishment rich in enzymes, vitamin C, essential fatty acids, minerals, amino acids and natural sugars.

Tomatoes: Stuffed with the powerful antioxidant lycopene, tomatoes have shown remarkable power to fight heart disease and cancer. Cooking tomatoes in oil helps your body absorb this antioxidant even better.

Yoghurt: Choose pots that contain live, active cultures to tackle yeast infections, lower cholesterol and prevent intestinal infections. Also a good source of minerals for happy, healthy bones.

> ★ **STAR BOX** *Wise up on your greens. The darker green the vegetable, the more vitamin C, beta-carotene, iron and calcium it contains.*

The little pills stars swear by

Supplements, vitamins, minerals and tinctures – celebrities take them all in the quest for a healthier and fitter body. If they've got a twinge, a cold or just want extra health insurance, here are the hottest natural remedies they swallow:

Chromium

The most important mineral for maintaining insulin function and controlling blood glucose. Some see this as a natural diet pill, as it is a co-factor in fat, protein and carbohydrate metabolism.

Co-enzyme Q10

An enzyme that plays an essential role in the release of energy from food. It is normally made in the body, but the ability to do so declines with age. It is most commonly taken to fight fatigue.

Conjugated Linoleic Acid

CLA inhibits the body's mechanism for storing fat and causes fatty reserves to be used for energy. Scientists have indicated that there is less CLA in our diet today than 30 years ago and believe this reduced intake could be a contributing factor to the steady rise in obesity.

Echinacea

Known to be a powerful immune-system booster, it is said to reduce the severity of cold and 'flu symptoms. Extensive studies have shown that it does increase the production of the white blood cells that destroy viruses.

Ginkgo Biloba

Most commonly taken to help improve short-term memory and maintain mental alertness.

Ginseng

The Chinese version of chicken soup. The purported benefits of ginseng include boosting your energy levels and immune system, helping with stress levels and improving your sex life!

Glucosamine

This occurs naturally in the joints and acts as the initial starting-block around which connective tissues, such as cartilage, tendons and ligaments, are built.

Grapeseed Extracts

Naturally found in berries, grapes, cherries and wine. 'A natural antioxidant, grapeseed extracts are important to skincare because they protect collagen from free radicals, dampen inflammation and help maintain the health and integrity of blood vessels,' Dr Perricone divulges. He recommends looking for reddish-purple capsules to be sure you're getting a concentrated natural supplement.

Green Foods

Read 'spiruliana, chlorella and wheat grass'. Achingly trendy, these have seen an upsurge of popularity, which primarily stems from the fact that these supplements are teeming with a wide array of vitamins, minerals, enzymes and highly digestible proteins. They are frequently used as detoxifiers and energy foods.

St John's Wort

The natural answer to Prozac. And with the stars as highly strung as they are, this supplement is seductive for its significant antidepressant effects.

Body shopping: when dieting isn't necessary

When the stars want to wriggle into a (very) little black dress and they've had enough of munching on cabbage leaves or sticking to juice fasts, they quite literally turn to a short cut to looking svelte and 'leaned out'. This is where their very discreet cosmetic surgeon's skills come into play. Whether it looks like it or not, many celebrities succumb to a little nip here and a little tuck there to improve their bodies, thinking of it as 'maintenance' therapy. And they're doing it sooner rather than later. In an age where celebrities – especially women of every age – are judged by their looks and more specifically the state of their bodies, surgery can give them a certain amount of control over their appearance in a short time period.

'Celebrities who "have it", generally have it. And the "in-betweens" are a wide range that can go from ordinary to stunning and often do so with a tummy tuck, breast implants and liposuction. If you are in the entertainment business, quick and frequent surgeries are the norm.'

Laurence Kirwan, *leading cosmetic surgeon*

Here Laurence Kirwan gives the low-down on procedure:

Liposuction

According to Kirwan this is now the most frequently performed aesthetic surgery procedure both in the USA and the UK. He says, 'Celebrities as well as normal women consider liposuction to smooth out their lumps and bumps from all those horrid areas which stubbornly remain less than svelte, especially around the hips, buttocks and outer thighs.' Liposuction literally means the removal of fat by suction and best results are obtained with the elastic skin of younger women. For her comeback movie, *Charlie's Angels: Full Throttle*, Demi Moore was rumoured in the tabloids to have had £240,000 worth of surgery, including liposuction on her stomach, buttocks and thighs.

Breast Implants

Up front and proud: great-looking breasts that are always jostling for attention are a leading woman's most wanted accessories. Despite all the bad press surrounding implants, firm and perky breasts are still longed for. Conscious of the fact that conventional breast augmentation is not appropriate for women with breasts that have become 'ptotic' (otherwise known as droopy), usually through childbirth, breastfeeding, weight loss or ageing, the breast option is a breast augmentation and mastopexy: the combination of implants along with an uplift. The excess skin is removed and the implant is placed to achieve the desired size. The advantage is it gives you everything at once!

Tummy Tuck

'This is called for when the abdominal muscles are stretched and the skin is loose,' explains Kirwan. 'The only cure is to tighten the muscles and remove the extra skin.' An incision that is hidden in a high-cut bikini bottom is made, the extra skin is removed, a new belly button is fashioned from the old one and the muscles are repaired.

Buttock Lift

'This will tighten the back of the thigh to a limited extent, but more importantly, it gives a nice curve to the buttock and removes any extra skin folds at the rear end of the buttock,' divulges Laurence, 'and it is the procedure for those who have had every possible ounce of fat suctioned and have lost any remaining body fat through exercise and diet.'

The Lower Body Lift

Kirwan describes this procedure as the most radical but also the most effective and portrays it as akin to 'pulling your pants up'! 'If you stand side-on in front of the mirror naked, grab the skin on one side of your hips at waist level and pull it upwards, this will create a tight upper thigh and buttock. This essentially is what the LBL achieves,' he says.

The Upper Body Lift

Developed by Kirwan, this procedure sounds the stuff B-list horror movies are made of: the surgeon cuts and tucks the skin along the crease under the breast and around the back to midline so the upper abdomen and back are flattened out, allowing for a smooth bodyline in dresses and swimsuits.

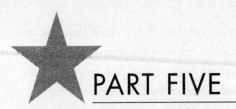 PART FIVE

Figuring it out the celebrity way

Let's get one thing straight: you don't bag an out-of-this-world body by sitting around on it. You may think Halle Berry was born with ready-toned Tinseltown arms and tight abs and was more than willing, ready and able to strip down to an itsy orange bikini in her role as a Bond girl without any body-sculpting help, but in reality she put the 'work' into her workouts. When you're paid to look good, taking care of your body is a full-time job.

For many women in the spotlight their body is their USP (Unique Selling Point) . And award ceremonies can be stars' biggest opportunity to make a lasting impression on the industry, along with countless millions of celebrity-hungry viewers. Red-carpet pictures are a permanent image. The upshot is, no screen siren wants to be seen as out of shape, worn out and desperate.

'The amount of pressure a star has to look just right is unimaginable. But although a better shape is a distinct advantage, it's not the only reason they work hard at working out. They actually want to be fit enough to keep up with their relentless schedules.'

Kathryn Freeland, *personal trainer*

Getting into shape in the first place is a tough business, which is why personal trainers are called upon. The star-shapers create bodies by design and the most wanted are part taskmaster, part caregiver, and great listener. Plus, they must be up on the latest in exercise physiology, sports medicine and nutrition. They must be dependable, discreet (no one likes their trouble spots being aired on daytime TV), creative and most importantly likeable, as a huge amount of time is spent up close and personal with the stars (in fact so personal Madonna had Lourdes with her trainer!)

'Jennifer Lopez is one of the hardest-working people I've ever met. Jennifer doesn't try to get out of anything, that's why she looks as incredible as she does.'

Gunnar Peterson, *celebrity personal trainer*

And the compliments are mutual. 'Gunnar's so knowledgeable about what it takes to get you burning calories,' says Lopez, who once said she could serve coffee using her rear as a ledge. 'He says a little bit of soreness is good. But not where you never want to come back.'

As for Angelina Jolie, whose athletic *Tomb Raider* body has been voted the most coveted physique in a patient survey run by The Beverly Hills Institute for Aesthetic and Reconstructive Surgery,

Gunnar describes her as a phenomenal person: 'Angelina Jolie is tireless. She's a gamer, that's what I would call her. She's ready for anything. You can take her through hard exercises, hard rep counts, slow cadence, whatever it is she's just right there with you.'

It's no surprise that the most wanted physiques are shapely, muscular bodies, and that means no space for slacking.

> 'In terms of motivation, I find that celebrity clients are a bit more motivated to facilitate change in their bodies because they realise that they are their own product.'
>
> **Michael George,** *personal trainer to Meg Ryan and Reese Witherspoon*

To keep you motivated to move and to fight off body boredom, I've rounded up a group of the most sought-after trainers with the most packed schedules, the most starry clientèle and the longest waiting lists to impart their tried and tested shape-you-up secrets.

★ **STAR BOX** *How you exercise has as much to do with your head as your body. Motivation has to be personal: if your partner is the reason you started shaping up in the first place, you're more likely to fail. It's people with personal motives who are more likely to achieve good results.*

Working out your body blueprint

Challenge any woman about her body shape and she invariably says she craves a trimmer waist, a tighter bum, sleeker thighs or simply less padding. Yet while every passing month brings a new faddy diet, the question of what truly determines each person's body shape is highly personal and how far it can be remoulded relies not solely on willpower but also on genetics. Unfortunately, no matter how hard you pray there is very little you can do to outwit the structure you were born with. There are certain things you can't change about your body. Bone structure is set for life and certain areas such as shoulders and hips are obviously more dependent on their bone for shape than fat or muscle.

'Don't set unrealistic goals for yourself. You have to look at the genetic hand you were dealt. So, if you have genetically wide hips, maybe you need to work the shoulders a little more to make sure they have adequate breadth to them, then you'll be surprised at how much smaller the behind looks.'

Gunnar Peterson

Gunnar's comments confirm that our bodies are all different, so all of us conforming to the same exercise regime doesn't make sense. If you're predisposed to having unfashionably placed fat cells or biggish bones, your workout is going to be different from that of a slim-hipped natural clothes-horse. The key is following an exercise programme designed to make the most of the body you were born with.

YOUR BODY BLUEPRINT
Body Blueprint: Very slim without much body fat
Celebrity Type: Calista Flockhart
Needs to: Follow a strength-training programme to create muscle mass and shape curves.
Ideal Regime: Start with a cardiovascular workout such as jogging twice a week for 20–30 minutes. This is not to solely burn fat, but to build up heart and lung fitness. Then include resistance work such as rowing, cycling or stepping to increase muscle mass. In addition, build up bone density and upper body strength by doing arm, chest and back exercises using light weights

(3–5lb), doing 8–12 reps and continuing to the point of muscle fatigue – as in 'I couldn't do another one!' If you're not using dumbbells, use the following gym machines: chest press, seat row and shoulder press

Danger Zone: If you're underweight, you have an increased risk of osteoporosis. Strength training will help with this, as will a diet high in calcium (milk, cheese, yoghurt and oily fish) to build up and maintain healthy bones.

Body Blueprint: The classic British pear.
Narrow shoulders, small waist, generous hips.
Celebrity Type: Kate Winslet

Needs to: Concentrate on strength training for the upper body and aerobic activity to whittle down an often troublesome lower body.

Ideal Body Workout: Make it your goal to fit in three aerobic sessions a week lasting from 30 to 60 minutes. If you can't make classes at the gym, try swimming, dancing or cycling, working at a low to moderate intensity. In addition, twice a week, slip in a 20 to 40-minute strength-training session to work the shoulders, back and chest. Defining and developing the muscles in these areas will help even out your bottom-heavy proportions.

Danger Zone: Don't go OTT on the Stairmaster. It will bulk up your bottom half. And remember, you may have a flat stomach, but your bottom and thighs are magnets for fatty foods. So drop the dessert!

Body Blueprint: Well-built with a tendency to being overweight

Celebrity Type: Liv Tyler

Needs to: Lose weight by reducing calorie intake and burning fat without bulking up.

Ideal Body Workout: Involves constant motion. Workout aerobically three to five times a week. Try brisk walking, cycling and circuit training, moving at a moderate pace and pushing yourself to the point of feeling fatigued. Start off with 20-minute sessions, gradually building up to 40 minutes or more. Twice a week after cardio training, tone the body with light resistance work, doing 12–18 reps for one set, then building up to two. Yoga and Pilates are good exercises for this body type as stretching helps to elongate the muscles for a more graceful shape.

Danger Zone: Avoid working out using heavy weights, as they'll build you up more. Take care when carrying out high-impact activities. Although it's tempting to burn off more calories, if you're overweight, your centre of gravity can shift, placing additional weight and unnecessary stress on joints.

★ **STAR BOX** *Become familiar with your body fat percentage as much as your weight and body type shape. Reducing body fat is an important first step to redefining your curves. The ideal body fat percentage for a female aged between 18 and 39 falls between 21 per cent and 33 per cent.*

Staying ahead of the curve: hip ways to exercise

In the words of personal trainer Kathy Kaehler, whose shape-me-up list is somewhat starry (Michelle Pfeiffer, Lisa Kudrow and Jennifer Aniston), 'Actors don't generally do well with boredom,' which is perhaps why they will trade in their run-of-the-mill aerobics class for something weird and wonderful. Fitness fads more often than not kick-start with the famous. So what the celebs get to grips with today can inspire you tomorrow.

'The problem is, if people get bored with their exercise regime, they stop doing it. If you can keep challenging them, it keeps them motivated,' concludes Kaehler.

And then there's the holistic side. 'I work on all three elements of self: emotional, spiritual and physical,' quips Kacy Duke, creative consultant to Manhattan's Equinox Fitness Clubs and personal trainer to Julianne Moore and Iman. 'When these three are in balance, that's a healthy body. I also encourage people to keep the body guessing.

It's like life – we don't do the same thing every day, so why should your workout be any different?' Which may go a little way towards explaining some of these exercise regimes with star appeal:

Star Exercise Turn: Pilates

If you haven't heard of Pilates you must have been on the moon eating cheese. It would be easier to list the celebrities who don't follow this exercise system. Developed in the 1920s and hailed as 'the thinking person's exercise', it's a discipline that improves flexibility and strength for the total body without the fear of bulking it up. Once you have absorbed the principles of Pilates, posture will improve, joints become mobile, muscles toned and the body balanced, elongated and poised. Not surprisingly, it has been the dancers' exercise secret for years and since been championed by Madonna and Courteney Cox, along with a host of other body beautifuls. When a nude scene in a movie is called for the stars always head straight for their Pilates studio, as they know it will get their bodies into really good shape.

Star Exercise Turn: Yogilates

A hybrid of yoga and Pilates and loved by Cate Blanchett, Yogilates, as the name suggests, combines the toning, flexibility and relaxation of yoga with the core strength and alignment of Pilates. Together they help build one lean body with super sexy, long, lean muscles.

Star Exercise Turn: Gyrotonics

An innovative exercise system that's already well established in New York and credited with shaping up Liv Tyler and Julianne Moore, gyrotonics involves a specially designed piece of equipment being built around the body and incorporates key principles of gymnastics, swimming, ballet and yoga. Described as 'moving meditation engaging the spirit as well as the anatomy' the machine gently releases energy blocks and encourages freedom of movement with exercises performed in circular and spiral motion.

Star Exercise Turn: Yoga

You name the celebrity, they do it! Meaning 'union of the body', yoga is so achingly hip it hurts. A workout for body and soul, it's the mother of all exercises when it comes to blissed-out joints and lean bodies. There's Bikram yoga, otherwise known as 'sweaty yoga', which is carried out in temperatures of 90° plus and said to be a favourite of Julia Roberts, Ashtanga yoga, a dynamic type of yoga and the one that got Madonna looking armed and dangerous, and Hypno-yoga, that is a combination of yoga and hypnosis-style meditation enjoyed by Cindy Crawford. All involve asanas, otherwise known as poses, that are said to release tension, increase energy and leave you feeling so very happy!

Star Exercise Turn: Cardio Striptease

Taking it off has certainly hit it off with some A-listers. Jennifer Aniston, Renée Zellweger and Carmen Electra are all said to have been mixing the art of striptease dancing with a cardiovascular workout at the trendy hangout that is Crunch Fitness. The latest in fashion fitness, it's said to be sensual, not sleazy, and promotes self-esteem, making women feel more comfortable with their bodies while at the same time toning them up. The one-hour classes include flirty gestures, sexy gyrations and graceful body caresses teamed with a low-impact exercise routine.

Star Exercise Turn: Boxercise

The stars have been quick to don their gloves and fight their way to top fitness. An action-packed fitness class that's been dubbed 'foxy boxing', boxercise incorporates a number of boxing moves and techniques without the physical contact. The only thing you punch is the bag and thin air. Fun, energetic and addictive, it's a great way of getting rid of that aggression when you lose out on parts. Hitting a heavy bag is similar to weight training in principle because it offers resistance and power moves that punch up your heart rate. Every hook and jab puts your stomach, waist and lower back to work and your arms and shoulders are exercised to give your upper body a toned look.

Star Exercise Turn: Krav Maga

As mentioned, if there's one star who pulls out all the stops when it comes to fitness it's Jennifer Lopez. To prepare for her role in *Enough*, she looked to Krav Maga and hung out for three months with an ex-LA policeman. The Israeli defence forces created this self-defence system before it was adopted by the American police. A tough combination of kick-boxing and circuit training, it teaches you how to defend yourself against common chokes, grabs, bearhugs and other attacks. Not for shrinking violets, this regime takes no prisoners and is slightly more aggressive than most martial arts. Headbutting and groin kicking are not unheard of. It's one hell of a shape-me-up.

The 5 Top Tips to Stick with It

1. Don't set yourself up for something so unrealistic that you're going to fail before you start. If you haven't been to the gym for the past five years, don't plan on going for the next 30 days straight.

2. Train with a gym buddy. It beats solo boredom and brings in a healthy level of competition.

3. Keep your programme short. All you need is 30 to 60 minutes, ideally three times a week.

4. Train where you feel comfortable and not simply because it's fashionable to be seen there. Most stars hook up with personal trainers so they don't have to sweat it out in a public gym!

5. Keep a training diary to track your progress. This ensures that you are improving your fitness levels. Seeing a jam-packed diary is a great motivator. After six months a complete re-evaluation of core goals will deliver new impetus.

Moves to look fashion fit

Forget best movie, best actress and even best director, there should be an Oscar for the actress with the best-toned body. A-list bodies generally have to be 100 per cent strong and sexy and unwrapped at a moment's notice. A flashgun-popping big-night-out dress rarely gives them the option of covering any areas they'd rather keep under wraps.

Personal trainer Simon Waterson is primarily known as the 007 trainer. Along with putting Bond himself, aka Pierce Brosnan, though fat-burning paces, he has also been called on set to whip the gorgeous Sophie Marceau, Denise Richards and Halle Berry, one of the best bodies in Hollywood, into shape. The mission? To guarantee they look fantastic enough to wear next to nothing while seducing Bond himself. So what's Simon's secret on getting celebrities into mega shape quickly?

'I'm into hard-core fitness. I haven't time for pampering celebrities' egos and for time-wasters who aren't prepared to work hard. When I take a client on I put them on a 10-week course and if they don't come up with the results, I resign them.'

Simon Waterson, *personal trainer to Halle Berry*

Tough talking indeed! And when it comes to working out, Simon sticks with his KIS principle. That means Keep It Simple. He says, 'I believe in developing a workout system that builds fitness fast and is completely adaptable. There's little doubt that Halle had a great body to begin with and my job was ultimately to give her that extra 10 per cent and sandpaper and buff her up around the edges for her scenes in *Die Another Day* to give her body a little more definition.'

So, whether you want to give yourself a total body workout or just fix a particular flaw, here are the session secrets used by top trainers on their famous clients to literally kick their arses into shape. They could just be the moves your body needs for the figure of your celluloid dreams.

★ **STAR BOX** *To maximise the number of calories burned in a single workout the answer is to cross train. Alternate between weight-training sets on the lower and upper body – for instance, chest flies would follow leg extensions. This forces the blood to all the extremities, revving your metabolism and burning more fat.*

LEAN AND LONGER-LOOKING LEGS

It doesn't matter if they're short or up to your armpits, fabulous legs are ones that are toned with lots of muscle definition. High-intensity strengthening exercises are the surest route to fit-to-be-seen pins, plus making a deal with yourself to put them to good use every day. Walking, cycling and swimming are all good daily leg toners, as these activities burn fat and tone the thighs and bottom without adding bulk. Be smart with your moves too. You can transform an exercise from one that strengthens to one that lengthens simply by adding an extra stretch to a classic move or holding a position for a second or two longer.

Pliés with Calf Raises

Stand with your legs hip-width apart, toes turned out, hands on your hips. Bend your knees until your thighs are almost parallel to the floor. Raise your heels up and down as many times as you can.

Inner Leg Lift

Flab often hits the inner leg first because these muscles aren't generally exercised during everyday activity.

Lie on your right side with your left leg crossed over your right and resting in front of you. Extend your right leg, keeping the knee slightly bent, and slowly lift it about one foot off the floor, using the inner thigh muscle to initiate the movement. Slowly lower your leg back down. Repeat 8–12 times for two sets.

Outer Thigh Raises

Toning the muscles on the outsides of your upper legs will help diminish any unsightly bulges.

Begin by lying on your right side with your bottom leg bent at a 45° angle. Extend your top leg out in front of you with the foot flexed. Keep your weight forward by leaning on your left hand (your hips should not roll backwards). Slowly lift your leg for a count of two, then lower for a count of two. Repeat as many times as comfortable.

FLAT AND AMAZING ABS

It's the season of the midriff every season as far as celebrities are concerned. A flat stomach is ultimately what every woman really wants and apart from making navel-gazing a whole lot more desirable, tight abs are key to a healthy and strong body. They're the core foundation to a healthy back, plus strong stomach muscles will help give your torso the stability and support necessary to protect your back from injury.

'The reason the abs are called a six pack is because they're six different muscles. I put my clients through six different abdominal moves in a session for the best results.'

Simon Waterson

Here are a few that get results:

Slow Crunches

Lie on your back with your knees bent and feet flat on the floor. Cross your arms across your chest, resting your right fingertips on your left shoulder and your left fingertips on your right shoulder. Using the muscles in your stomach, slowly raise your torso off the floor until your elbows touch your thighs. Hold for one second. Then resume your starting position. Do three sets of 10 to 15 reps.

The Plank

'This is a yoga-inspired move I advised Cate Blanchett to do. She hated doing it but it's so effective to get rid of a lower tummy bulge.'

Kathryn Freeland, *personal trainer*

Position yourself so that your toes are on the ground and your elbows are directly below your shoulders. Raise yourself up, keeping a straight line from your shoulders to your ankles, so that your elbows and toes support your body. Pull in your abdominal muscles and don't let your bottom stick in the air. Hold for as long as possible – for instance, a minute.

Abdominal Circles

Lie on your back with your knees bent, feet flat to the floor and hip-width apart. Support your head with your hands but don't pull your head forwards. Tuck your chin under slightly and pull your abs in tight towards your spine. Lift your head, neck and shoulder blades off the floor and hold. Make a small circle with your waist clockwise heading left, across the top to the right and down. This is one circle. Repeat five times in each direction.

BETTER BREASTS ON SHOW

Forget the idea that great-looking breasts are all fake. They're not. The most popular A-listers' are all natural: Cameron Diaz, Jennifer Aniston and Gwyneth Paltrow. They just make the most of what God dished out to them. Exercise won't change the actual shape or size of your breasts, as there are no muscles in them to tone and lift – it's all fat and glands – but what zone-specific exercises will do is strengthen and tone the surrounding pectoral muscles: the underlying fan-shaped muscles around the breasts.

Chest Flies

Grab a 5lb (2.5kg) weight in each hand and lie on your back with your knees bent, feet flat on the floor and arms bent so that your knuckles are touching your shoulders. Press the weights towards the ceiling until your arms are straight with the palms facing each other. Lower the weights out to each side at the same time until you feel a stretch in the chest. Resume the original position. Do 10 reps for two sets.

Chest Presses

Stand holding a 5lb (2.5kg) weight in each hand with your arms by your sides. Keeping your elbows still, bend your arms so that the weights come to shoulder height, with your palms facing forwards. Next, fully extend your arms in front of your body, keeping your back straight and stomach muscles pulled in. Then bend them again. Do two sets of 10 without lowering the weights in between movements.

Pullovers

Lie on your back with your knees bent and feet flat on the floor. Put your arms straight behind your head so your elbows graze your ears, with a 5lb (2.5kg) weight in your hands. Keeping your arms straight, raise the weight off the floor until your hands are directly above your chest (not your face). Resume the starting position. Do two sets of 10 reps.

ARMS WITH ATTITUDE

Celebrities do not do arms that wave long after their hands have stopped. Tight triceps and buffed biceps are where it's at. Flabby chicken wings are not an option!

The dumbbell is seen as the fastest route to sexy arms, although most women avoid free weights for fear of bulking up. 'Not true,' says Gunnar Peterson. 'You're going to burn fat by strength training. Women tend to worry that lifting weights will make them bulk up, but the truth is, weights don't make you big. Food does.'

Overhead Tricep Extensions

To hit flabby underarms, sit upright on a chair with your back straight and feet flat on the floor. Hold a 5lb (2.5kg) dumbbell with your left hand behind your head and down between your shoulder blades. Extend your arm, keeping the weight close to your body and elbow pointing upwards. Don't let your elbow wander and keep your abdominal muscles tight to prevent straining your back. Slowly return to the starting position. Repeat with your right arm, doing two sets of 12 reps.

Shoulder Presses

Although pleasing arms need firm biceps and triceps, shoulder definition also helps shape them. Here's a move to work the shoulders.

Sit on a chair with your back well supported and legs bent at 90°. Hold a 5lb (2.5kg) dumbbell in each hand and with your arms bent at 90° and elbows out at shoulder level. Press the weights upwards, raising your arms above the head. Do not lock your arms straight. Pause briefly, then breathe in as you lower the weights to shoulder height. Repeat 12 reps for two sets.

Rotating Hammer Curls

To tone the biceps, stand up straight with your feet together and a 5lb (2.5kg) dumbbell in each hand. Keep your arms by your sides. Bending your elbow, slowly curl the left dumbbell towards your left shoulder. Be sure to keep your elbow close to your body. As you lower your left arm back to the starting position, rotate the dumbbell as if you were about to use it as a hammer. Repeat with the right arm to complete one rep. Repeat 12 times on each arm for two sets.

A BUFFED-UP BUTT

Bottoms seduce, but unfortunately the buttocks are where women's bodies are biologically predetermined to store excess fat, so toning this area can be a little tougher than other parts of the body. The most effective way to burn fat around the hips and bottom is to work the body aerobically and throw in exercise targeted to increase muscle use and fat reduction in those areas. One of the major causes of a bottom sliding southwards is leading a sedentary lifestyle. So get off it and start moving it! Brisk walking, cycling or dancing are all incidental ways you can firm it up.

Walking Lunges

Lunges are done by A-listers everywhere. They are not only good for balance and co-ordination, but really shape up your bottom double quick. Stand with your feet hip-width apart and your knees slightly bent. Put your hands on your hips. Step forwards about one stride length from your back foot. In the same movement, lower your body down, hold for one second then, raising your body, step forwards with the other leg and repeat the lunge. Continue as you move forwards for 30.

The Weighted Squat

Holding a 5–8lb (2.5–3.5kg) weight in each hand, stand upright with your feet parallel and shoulder-width apart. Keep your abs and buttocks tense. Lower yourself into a sitting position as you would on a chair. Hold for one second. As you rise, squeeze your buttocks. Repeat 12 times for two sets.

The Duke Curtsey

This is a move Kacy Duke uses on Iman and Julianne Moore. Standing upright with your abs tight and your hands on your waist, heels and toes turned out slightly, in a single fluid movement bring your right leg back and towards the left side, bending both knees into a curtsey while keeping your back straight. Return to the starting position and repeat 12 times before changing to your left leg.

A Blade-baring Rear View

For every bewitching entrance there has to be a sexy exit. And with dresses becoming ever more daring, the unwrapped back has become the fastest new erogenous zone. Although Jamie Lee Curtis admitted to having 'back fat', many A-listers would rather exercise away their bra-strap bulge than bypass the photo opportunity of showing off a strong and sculptured rear view in a sexy cutaway number. As far as Hollywood is concerned, bottom cleavage is here to stay!

Shoulder Lifts

Sit on the edge of a chair with 5lb (2.5kg) weights in each hand. Keeping your arms by your sides, bend at the waist until your chest touches your thighs. Without bending your arms, raise them out to each side until they are shoulder level. Slowly lower. Do 10 reps for three sets.

Shrugs

Stand with your feet shoulder-width apart, your knees slightly bent. Hold a 5lb (2.5kg) dumbbell in each hand, your palms facing your thighs. Exhale, lifting your shoulders to your ears. Hold for one count. Return to the start, inhaling for a count of three. Do 20 reps for three sets.

Back Raises

Lie face down with your legs extended and your feet together. Stretch your arms over your head. Pull your abs in and press your hips into the floor. Breathe out as you raise your right arm and left leg to a comfortable height. Hold briefly at the top of the movement, then breathe in as you slowly return your arm and leg to the floor. Repeat using your right leg and left arm. Repeat 20 reps on each side for three sets.

'Don't rush your body-shaping moves. Slowing down and concentrating on the exercise makes it extremely effective.'

Simon Waterson

Première secrets: how to get a better body for that dress!

As you've guessed by now, looking resplendent on the most-photographed rug takes time and work. The most-wanted fitness trainers are not too dissimilar to great directors: they emphasise that the only way to a body licensed to thrill is to follow a finely tuned fitness script. And its three acts are: part one: stay in reasonable shape all year round; part two: eat small and frequent balanced meals; and part three: vary your exercise so your body doesn't fall into the comfort zone. But although these rules seem simple enough to follow, celebrities, like everyone else, can drop by the wayside. In the two weeks before the Oscars, trainers' phones are on meltdown from people who dared not follow the script and are in need of a body miracle. But although dropping 3–4lb (1–2kg) in 14 days is reasonable enough, any more and they're in trouble and looking to wear something a little less than skintight.

Gunnar Peterson says if you're not on a serious

programme a month before the big occasion you have to be realistic about your goals: 'You should be doing three days a week of cardiovascular work – at least 30 minutes a session – along with at least two days of strength training.' He advises a 'clean' diet with foods such as green vegetables and avoiding the heavier starches, plus adequate rest. For the two weeks prior to the big event Peterson says no more alcohol or desserts. 'Relax, it's only for a couple of weeks,' he says.

As the days go by, the stars become more focused. One week before the big showdown, Gunnar advises adding 15 minutes to each workout session and for the first four days of this week, no more complex carbohydrates after 5 p.m. On the day itself, eat no complex carbohydrates after 11 a.m. and eat a small meal before you head out. This will stop you keeling over after your first sip of champagne!

When it comes to instant pre-party pert and toning tips Simon Waterson knows the moves to make your body look leaner and meaner. Simon says it's arms and legs that everybody notices, especially as party dresses invariably have spaghetti straps and high-split skirts. And I'm listening – he does train Bond girls!

'You need to force blood into muscles which will be on display to give them a firm and curvy shape. Just before you slip on your dress, do three sets of 15 repetitions of tricep dips for the back of the arms, press-ups and lunges. Guys do press-ups if they want to seduce, so why shouldn't you?'

Simon Waterson

BEAT THE PRE-PARTY TUMMY BLOAT

It's enough to make an A-lister weep. Yesterday her tummy was as flat as a pancake and today it looks pumped up and fit to burst. A-lister or not, everyone is susceptible to tummy bloat and there's little doubt that it steals away body confidence. Whatever the cause of belly bulge – and it's not a lack of crunches when I'm talking about stars – it can leave a woman feeling low and unattractive. And there's one item of clothing that a star doesn't want to be photographed in on an all-eyes-on-me-night and that's trousers with an elasticised waistband. Here are tips on banishing the dreaded bloat:

★ Drink lots of water. The more H_2O you take in, the less your body will retain.

★ Cut out caffeine. It stimulates the intestine, causing it to contract and produce gas.

★ Skip the soda, including sparkling water. Remember what happens when you shake a can of soda and then open it fast? The drink sprays out because of the pressure. The same happens inside your stomach.

★ Don't chew gum. It causes you to swallow air and bloat.

★ Stop speed eating. You're not in a race. When you eat food quickly you gulp down air.

★ Avoid gas-causing foods. The obvious suspects are cabbage, Brussels sprouts and beans!

★ Relax. Stress makes the stomach overproduce acid that interferes with digestion, forcing undigested food into the intestine. This is feasted on by bacteria, which give off gas and cause bloating.

> ⭐ **STAR BOX** *When inch loss is called for, and fast, stars are not immune to mummifying themselves in body wraps. It may only be a Cinderella solution, but they can tighten up saggy skin something wonderful.*

The modern (Ma)donna: shape beyond pregnancy

'You look fabulous,' said my midwife after I gave birth to my son. Fact: I looked far from fabulous, but it's a compliment that every new mother wants to hear. Especially one in the limelight. Demi Moore made pregnancy 'fashionable' when posing naked on the front of *Vanity Fair* and paved the way for embracing celebrity pregnancies. Far from being sidelined, pregnant stars now flaunt their bare and swollen bellies with abandonment and post birth are put on a golden pedestal by the worldwide media as 'having it all': cutesome baby, success and a slim and sexy figure to boot. Catherine Zeta Jones even took to slipping into a black basque rather than hide away in Bridget Jones-style pants for the cover of *Vanity Fair* just 11 weeks after the birth of her son Dylan. And the mother of them all, Madonna, quipped: 'I don't want to sound immodest, but I don't think having a child has made me unsexy. There's nothing sexier than a mother.' And she thanked breastfeeding, power yoga, walking and cycling for dropping her baby pounds just two months after giving birth.

The pressure on women to zip themselves back into their jeans once they've left the maternity ward is enormous, and never more so than on a famous mum. In the figure-obsessed world that is Hollywood there are no jobs for lumpy, dumpy and frumpy-looking mums. Or, as quickly slimmed down Elizabeth Hurley said after the arrival of Damian, 'Being able to squeeze myself into tiny clothes is how I earn my living. Losing the weight was mostly iron will. I made it my mission to get back into shape.' Her post-Damian diet was reported to be watercress soup, steamed fish, brown rice and wheat-free oatcakes.

....

CELEBRITY PICKINGS *Celebrity fitness trainer Kacy Duke, who whipped mother-of-two Julianne Moore into shape, reveals that baby push-ups can be great for an at-home upper-arm flab fighter. 'Lie on the floor, with knees bent, and hold your baby an inch (2.5cm) above the chest. Extend arms up, hold for one second, return to the starting position. Do sets of eight repetitions,' she says.*

....

With rumours abounding of early Caesareans to stop the foetal pounds piling on and tummy tucks along with C-sections, take comfort that not all celebrities hold court two months post mini me in a Versace dress. Kate Winslet struggled to lose the four stone she put on with her baby, claiming, 'My bottom looked like purple sprouting broccoli, other body parts resembled squashes. I was an absolute sight, I really was.' Desperate to dump the post-birth bump and worried she would not get major parts without slimming down, Kate turned to facial analysis – a method of reading nutritional deficiency by looking at the face. By cutting out bread, dairy and red meat, Kate gradually shifted her weight gain and now she's back in the celluloid running.

Looking together, sexy and outright fabulous just days within giving birth may be part and parcel of being famous, but for normal mums it can give rise to anxiety and too much exercise too soon. It's very rare that we naturally snap back into shape after labour, as many of the pounds gained during the nine months are still stored in the body's cells and won't be lost until months after the event. However, there is no reason why you can't regain your figure, or even improve on it.

'Take it easy and you will reap the long-term rewards,' says Pilates expert Lynne Robinson, who was initially credited for getting Liz Hurley back into her high-style signature-style dresses just months after having her son. Liz got to grips with the principles of Pilates twice a week.

'You must wait six weeks after the birth before recommencing exercise. Elizabeth didn't even do one curl up until around the five-month mark as she had a Caesarean. The key thing to work on after giving birth is your stability and not flinging yourself around. Pelvic floor exercises are the secret to getting back your figure – and lots and lots please!'

Lynne Robinson, *Pilates teacher to Liz Hurley*

Exercises the stars love out of the gym

Atoned and lithe body doesn't all have to be Pilates and treadmill-based. The all-play workout can be just as effective as a super-quick shape-me-up programme. Incidental fitness – that's unplanned gym-free activities – is seriously underrated and can work your body harder than you think. Here are what the stars are into in their spare time.

Star: Renée Zellweger
Star Turn: Running. Whether it's to escape the prying lenses of the paparazzi or just to keep fit, Renée has found a reason to crank up her pace and run. Apart from giving you heaps more energy, sky-high endurance levels and a firmer and higher butt, running is great for the heart, acts as a weight-bearing activity which boosts bone density, and burns calories. Lots of them. In half an hour 450 calories are eaten right up. Thirty minutes a day, four days a week will give an excellent level of fitness in the shortest possible time. A programme of alternating running and walking

(otherwise known as 'interval training') is a good way to begin.

Star: Julia Roberts

Star Turn: Horseriding. Adventurous, exciting and fun, even gentle hacking burns up an impressive 40 calories per minute – that's 240 calories an hour. Plus horseriding places demands on the whole of the body and will exercise muscles in the legs, back and arms. Riding at a brisk trot for half an hour will challenge your whole cardiovascular system.

Star: Catherine Zeta Jones

Star Turn: Golf. Often seen as a sport for retired bank managers wearing dodgy jumpers, in reality golf makes an ideal exercise for all age groups and has been readily embraced by the Hollywood set. Along with Catherine, Sharon Stone, Cindy Crawford and Charlize Theron all hit the fairways. Swinging your club works on mobility, flexibility and strength in the arms, shoulders and back. Plus it's great for posture and all those swings make for a fine waist whittler, along with burning around 125 calories in half an hour.

Star: Madonna

Star Turn: Cycling. Who would have thought Mrs Ritchie would readily shed all the trappings of her celebrity life and so eagerly trade her chauffeur-driven cars for a ride in the saddle? Not only does cycling guarantee a quick getaway, it also burns calories. Riding at 10mph for an hour will burn off 240 calories and at 17mph for an hour will effortlessly eat up 720 calories. It's also great for leaner-looking legs, strength and stamina levels.

Star: Jennifer Aniston
Star Turn: Power walking. Walking is one of the most effective forms of exercise you can do and power walking can improve your fitness levels as fast as jogging, with the same speeds being gained without the heavy impact on the joints. It also means you can sustain the effort more easily at a moderate intensity for longer. It's been reported that walking up to four times a week for 45 minutes (that's less than your lunch hour) can reward you with a loss of 18lbs (8kg) a year without even changing your diet. Aim to walk fast enough so you can't hold a conversation, and carry water to avoid dehydration, taking small and frequent sips.

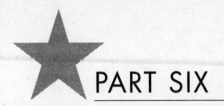

PART SIX

Dare to act like a diva

What does it take to be a diva? A gay following? Excessive late-ness? A fleet of limos? Or just falling into the habit of over-demanding and expecting?

Acting diva-ish is nothing new. Old-timers such as Marlene Dietrich, Joan Crawford, Bette Davis and Elizabeth Taylor had high maintenance down to a fine art. Today it's Mariah Carey and Jennifer Lopez who reportedly throw hissy fits and make outra-geous dressing-room demands. While in London promoting a film it was said that Jennifer's diva-like demands included that her plush hotel room should be decorated with white lilies, white linen, lemon-scented candles and white curtains. Hotel staff were not permitted to talk to her, all food had to be left out in the hall, only Cristal champagne was to be served and sushi and chocolate cake were to be available at all times. According to a 'source', 'As long as everything goes smoothly, then she's happy. But if it goes wrong, she can be prickly.'

One has to wonder what makes a famous person become so demanding. Read 'spoilt'. Do they feel they've earned the right or is it just the deadly combination of money and power? Whatever it is, their egos know no shame. And their requests are becoming

ever more bizarre and ridiculous. Mariah Carey for instance
'doesn't do stairs' and is said only to drink tea made with Poland
Spring water. Mariah explains: 'I know I can be diva-ish sometimes, but I have to be in control. The nature of my life, the nature
of what I do, is divadom, it really is.'

For an all-out celebrity attitude, I'm not telling you to start
stomping your foot like a three-year-old if the Evian isn't served
chilled, but how to turn heads in a room by walking the walk and
talking the talk. To really light up a room celebrity-style takes more
than fabulous hair and make-up: it takes genuine charisma and
know-how. But every woman can create her own allure. Sexual
confidence will come with great posture, and personal style
doesn't have to come with a hefty price tag – it's just knowing
how to throw it all together that matters. Make people hang onto
your every word – using the erotic power of your voice, of course
(a high pipsqueak should only be for mice). Finally, there's the
spin. A celebrity is never out of work, she's just 'resting'.
Celebrities have a knack of spinning their lives to their own advantage. You can too. You just have to learn how to spin with the
best of them – only faster!

Strike a pose: moves to a great posture

'Anytime I can look taller, I'm happy.'

Jennifer Aniston

And that's where great posture can come in. Who said there's no such thing as an instant makeover? Standing tall can add at least one to two inches (3–5cm) to your height as well as making it look as if you've lost a few pounds. On the other hand, there's nothing less sexy than a woman who hunches. Gwyneth Paltrow has been picked up many times by the press for lazy posture and some pictures make her look anything but a bona fide A-lister. Fact: dropping into yourself like Gwyneth can actually make you look miserable and dumpy, as your shoulders are permanently slumped forwards, making your neck look shorter.

'Elizabeth Hurley has great posture, which alone gives her amazing presence.'

Lynne Robinson, *Pilates teacher to Elizabeth Hurley*

Celebrities with instantly programmed posture include Catherine Zeta Jones and Sarah Jessica Parker – both trained dancers. Perfect poise can be a performance in itself.

ANATOMY LESSONS

Think of posture as a silent weapon in your image management and you'll never slump again. Posture works as an excellent looks enhancer and affects how other people see you. Plus it's a powerful performance booster. And be warned: those with a bad stance will never have thin-looking thighs. Each part of the body affects the next. As the upper part of the torso sinks down onto the lower part so the extra weight settles down onto the upper thighs.

The true power stance – standing upright with your shoulders relaxed and your upper body face onto the world – sends out strong messages that you're no pussycat (only when you want to be!) Here's how standing taller highlights different parts of the body:

Head: With the head weighing in at 15–20 lbs (5.6–9kg) it's all too easy to slump it forwards. Keep it held high. Not only will you look and feel taller, but a more defined jawline will reveal itself too. Imagine a balloon gently lifting you up from the top of your head.

Chin: Keep it tucked in. This means your head is sitting on top of your shoulders and not jutting arrogantly forwards, causing stress to neck joints and the upper back.

Neck: Position it so that your ears line up above your shoulders and hips.

Torso: If you slump forwards your waist goes AWOL. But

as you stretch upwards and separate the area between the ribcage and pelvis, it looks a whole lot slimmer and shapelier.

Shoulders: Keep them level, slightly back and pulled down from the ears. Do not wear your shoulders as earrings. If you pull your shoulder blades back, your arm muscles get improved definition and look altogether more toned.

Bust: Saggy-looking boobs can be put down to an ill-fitting bra or poor posture. Help lift the breasts by lengthening your spine and pulling your shoulder blades back.

Thighs: Slumping into a figure of depression can make your hips flabby, as the muscles around that area aren't given the chance to work to their full potential.

Bottom: Keep it tucked under rather than sticking it out. Crossing your legs twists your pelvis into an unnatural position and can cause lower back problems and affect posture. Cross your ankles instead.

WAYS TO GRAB SOME BACKBONE CHIC

Ears centred over shoulders, shoulders over hips, hips over knees and knees over ankles . . . it all sounds so darn simple, but nurturing good posture can be difficult after years of slouching. Still, you can't practise being a sexy diva if you don't know how to carry yourself.

Perfect alignment is all about learning the architecture of the body and how you can build on it. Balancing a book on top of your head won't give you better posture, but along with Pilates and yoga one of these programmes or specialists may coax your body out of its bad habits and into better alignment.

The Alexander Technique

A tailor-made teaching programme where the idea is to make good posture second nature. The teacher will help you unlearn your patterns of tension through verbal and hands-on guidance, helping you to relearn your body's optimum way of graceful and effortless moving.

Hellerwork

Deep reaching, restructuring and rebalancing bodywork, Hellerwork concentrates on de-hunching the body and freeing the negative emotions that can constrain it. Manipulation can be painful, but stick with the course and you'll be rewarded with added height and a straighter skeleton.

Chiropractor

A chiropractor is a spinal specialist. Rapid, forceful but painless movements are central to chiropractic treatment. Chiropractors frequently use X-rays to detect imbalances and muscle tension, and spasms can be quickly released for better posture and health.

★ **STAR BOX** *Do you ever see a diva lugging around a huge bag? No. That's because heavy bags can encourage scoliosis – curvature of the spine. To avoid lopsided shoulders, lighten the load and downsize your bag.*

How to walk in diva-like heels – without tripping

When it comes to soul searching, a diva will think 'sole searching' and look no further than a shoe shop. High heels maketh the woman and, ignoring the fact they're bad for your posture and your feet (oh, add podiatrist to the entourage), a well-worn pair of heels will emphasise every natural curve on a diva's body. Plus if she's not in the supermodel league when it comes to height, heels instantly add on a confidence-building four inches (10cm) or so. It's a well-known fact that when Nicole Kidman split from the much shorter Tom Cruise she said, 'Now I can wear heels.'

> 'When it comes to his heels, they are as good as sex – and they last longer.'
>
> **Madonna** *on Manolo Blahnik heels*

So what's the difference between wearing flats and heels? Flats are what traffic wardens wear, not divas, and they can have you walking like a carthorse. Heels in comparison bring out your inner sex kitten. Gucci, Prada, Gina and Jimmy Choo shoes are all lusted after by A-listers, as they are so well cut they bless the leg with a sexy high-arched line. And then there's Manolo Blahnik. Say: Ma-NO-low BLAH-nik. Sarah Jessica Parker has had the diva-ish privilege of having a Manolo shoe named after her: the Sarah Jessica. She explains: 'I think a high heel is one of the prettiest things imaginable. And as a short person – I'm 5 ft 4in – I count on a nice heel.'

Heels may look great, but walking in them gracefully is an art form in itself. The key word is *glide.* Not plod. The first point is to take small steps. Slow down and shorten your stride. Come down on the ball of your foot when you step. Do not walk on your heels but on your toes, keeping them pointing straight ahead or as close to straight ahead as possible.

For a catwalk walk red-carpet style, the secret is to overlap your feet as you walk by placing one foot in front of the other as opposed to walking with your feet side by side. This motion will look elegant and lend your hips an extra sway, making your dress or skirt move teasingly around your thighs.

Another A-lister tip is to visualise a hand pushing into the small of your back, just above your coccyx. This will give the desired effect of tilting your shoulders back and your chest forward.

As for what to do with your arms, let them hang loose, leaving your hands to trail an inch or two (2.5–5cm) behind your body.

When tackling stairs, make sure sole and heel land together firmly and simultaneously on each step. When descending stairs, only the sole of the shoe needs to hit each step.

> ★ **STAR BOX** *Avoid walking on ice, slush, mud, grass, gravel and other uneven surfaces. Slipping or sinking is not a good look. When in doubt, simply slip off your heels and elegantly carry them across such potential pitfalls in your bare (manicured) feet.*

Shop like a stylist, look like a star

Celebrities are clotheshorses as much as anything else. Designers know this only too well, which is why they are tripping over themselves to dress them. It's called 'celebrity endorsement'. Fashion houses know that an A-lister wearing one of their gowns will probably sell them more clothes and put them on the fashion map faster than a full-page ad placed in one of the top glossy magazines.

When it comes to gowning up for the Oscars or any other prestigious evenings, stylists are called in. Stars cannot be trusted to style themselves. Remember the disaster that was Kim Basinger when she designed her own satin dress at the Oscars? Most fashion houses have people or a public relations department that take care of the stars. This person is always in touch with the celebrity stylist so that when the gown-hunting is on, they know what to offer in the hope of getting their creations on the red carpet.

But, like everything else, get it right and you look fabulous, get it wrong and you could wind up looking like a dog's dinner and doing the designer more of a disservice than a favour. Remember the fashion horror of the white tuxedo jacket worn back to front on Celine Dion? When a star puts her heels on the red carpet, she hopes the dress will be a hit. If not, sack the stylist! This leads to the question: if a star has help throwing clothes together and still gets it wrong, what hope is there for civilians (as Elizabeth Hurley refers to the likes of you and me)? Quite a lot actually. Becoming a savvy shopper takes a trained eye, but once focused, a great wardrobe can come effortlessly together.

DRESSING TO THRILL

What's the secret to commanding hundreds of flashguns to go off together just to capture a life of dress? Here are a few well-hung clues:

★ Know your assets. Halle Berry, Julia Roberts and Catherine Zeta Jones all wriggle into slinky dresses to show off their well-honed figures. Whether it's your bust, waist or legs that are your favourite asset, choose an outfit that will show off your strong points to the max.

★ The LBD (little black dress) can be a girl's best friend. Forget the low-calorie diet. A good LBD is an instant slimmer and can be a crafty tool to minimise a generous bum. Jennifer Aniston and Julia Roberts do the LBD look so well. Keep it simple with décolletage drama and trade in a very short hemline (that can look a little tacky) for one that drops to the floor for sophisticated slinkiness.

★ Dump the fancy details like sequins, tiers of tulle and layers of ruffles if you don't want to look like the fairy on top of the Christmas tree.

★ Clutch an evening bag. A tote and a cocktail dress do not make for a streamlined look.

★ Keep your jewellery sparkling.

★ Wear skyscraper heels (see above on how to walk).

THE FIGURE FIXERS: SHAPES TO FLATTER YOUR BODY

It's been reported that J-Lo has all her size 10 labels in her clothes removed by her entourage and replaced with a size 6. Who knows if this bizarre piece of gossip is true? But what I do know is celebrities are as insecure about their bodies as the next person and needs to hide and disguise areas of their bodies they're not too hot about. They're only human, after all.

Sizing Yourself Up: Your Perfect Shape-enhancing Pieces

Figure Type: Curvy

Celebrity: Jennifer Lopez

Dress Code: This shape is not about hiding your figure, it's about showing it off. And J-Lo sure knows how to do this to maximum effect. First off, a plunging neckline takes the eye away from the hips and draws it up top. Marilyn Monroe, who boasted an hourglass figure, was in little doubt about this fashion secret. Secondly, a halter-neck top gives the illusion of extending the shoulder line and therefore balancing out the hips. Take a style tip from Jennifer and wear tight jeans. They look sexy on a toned booty. Keep things simple around the bottom area. Pockets and frills from the waist down will only emphasise your hips. For sleeves, go for sleeveless or full length. Capped sleeves can accentuate larger arms. And as for fabrics, keep them light and wispy. Heavy fabrics can make this figure look dumpier.

Figure Type: Petite
Celebrity: Madonna
Dress Code: Big in personality, small in body, Madonna never vanishes into the background. Vertical pinstripes look great on a smaller figure and give the illusion that you're taller than you actually are. Fitted single-breasted jackets look great too, buttoned up with nothing worn underneath. In fact the more fitted the cloth, the better. Swathing yourself in lots of loose fabric swallows up a small figure. Three-quarter sleeves are perfect for a petite frame too. Avoid decorating yourself with lots of trinkets. Once again, keep it simple and you will reap the fashion awards.

Figure Type: Tall
Celebrity: Julia Roberts
Dress Code: 'I'm too tall to be a girl. I'm between a chick and a broad,' states Julia Roberts. If unconfident, it can take a while for your personality to catch up with an above-average height. But as Julia Roberts, Liv Tyler and Sigourney Weaver know, there's something very sexy and powerful about being tall. Make your height

your asset by wearing trousers with tapered legs, opt for soft and sensual fabrics that drape the body and wear V-necklines. They show off a graceful neck, so play it up with linear earrings – a favourite look of Nicole Kidman. Polo necks also look good on a longer torso, and for prints, keep them small to balance your figure. Don't wear anything cropped – it can make you look thick-waisted. Also avoid layering – it can add unwanted bulk to your frame.

Figure Type: Thin
Celebrity: Calista Flockhart
Dress Code: Being thin can have its fashion problems too. Anything baggy is a definite no-no, as in long flowing layers. The idea is to add femininity and create curves. This is one body shape that can carry off ruffles and patterns to give the impression of a fuller figure. Slip skirts and wraparound dresses look great, as do Capri-style straight-leg trousers – a look perfected by Audrey Hepburn. A word on dresses: a very low-cut dress can highlight a bony chest and make you look flatter than you actually are. Layering works well. Mix it up – this figure gives the opportunity to experiment. It can make patterns married with stripes married with spots look stylish and kooky.

Wear It Well and Drop 5lb (2.5kg)

When it comes to celebrity style, the basic principles are to let fashion flatter your shape. Stylists and personal shoppers have learned that small prints, too many colours and shiny fabrics are a fuller figure's downfall. Why? Well, for starters, just as large prints can swamp petite figures, so fiddly patterns can make generous shapes look even more ample. And the secret of colour is wising up to the fact that hot attention-grabbing hues such as reds, yellows and oranges can all expand. Cool shades such as blues, green, browns and blacks all give the magical effect of shrinking a larger shape down a dress size or two.

Now for a word on texture. To effortlessly melt pounds away, one should turn a blind eye to big cuddly jumpers in bulky knits, crisp and starchy cotton and heavy fabrics for suiting. Instead fabrics should be kept light and soft – wool, crepes, linens and silks. These fabrics look and feel sensual, as well as giving a leaner shape.

Now the basic rules have been set, let's get down to some shopping logic. Starting from the neck down, it's a fact that although small-busted girls may well envy those more generously endowed, it's usually the woman with a fuller bust who often sheds tears in the dressing room. The fluid line of a shirt, dress or jacket can be ruined by a large bust. The answer is to go for tailored dresses, shirts and tops. Salma Hayek knows this all too well. To prevent button-holes from straining, the trick is to take a bigger size than normal. But don't worry, the tailoring will help slenderise so you won't wind up looking a size bigger.

To slim down bottoms, thighs, hips and legs, stylists stake out clothes that do all the hard work for the stars. For hips, the secret is to draw attention to your upper half. V-neck tops and ruffles all draw the eye nicely upwards. Avoid jackets, shirts or sweaters that finish on the broadest curve of your hips. To disguise a thick waist, opt for unstructured shapes, and by this I don't mean smocks but modern-cut tunics worn over trousers for elegance. If wearing a belt, wear it loose. If it moves, it gives the illusion of extra room. Keep away from gathered or drawstring skirts and trousers, all of which enlarge the waistline to uncelebrity proportions.

Closet Encounters: Smart Wardrobe Tactics

★ Wear straight silhouettes if you have a thick waist. Anything nipped in will draw attention to it.

★ To lengthen short legs, opt for slim-fit cigarette pants or dresses that hit the knee. Wear with a pointy mule or heel.

★ Horizontal stripes create width, diagonal stripes give a fluid look. And the skinnier the stripe, the thinner you will appear.

★ Swap suits for dresses. The more lines and seams you have, the less attention is drawn to lumps and bumps underneath.

★ Boot-leg cut trousers with a slight flare at the bottom make your thighs appear thinner.

★ Hide a tummy with flat-front trousers that flatten you all around. Don't even consider front-pleated trousers.

★ For a large bust, don't wear a keyhole neckline. There's no support and it can look vulgar. Go for a higher, wider neckline.

Words from a Master of Style

When the stars want to pull out all the stops they call Phillip Bloch, Hollywood's premier stylist, whose client list reads like *Who's Who*: Sandra Bullock, Salma Hayek and Faye Dunaway. Phillip readily admits that when dressing a star for a big event he always has the paparazzi in mind and looks for a 'press dress' for maximum impact. In fact such a style authority has he become that he's written a book entitled *Elements of Style* with great Hollywood advice for everyday people. Here are his rules for looking better than your rival:

Necklines: 'The right neckline should frame your face beautifully and bare as much or as little as you're comfortable showing. A draped neckline is an elegant way to show deep cleavage without somehow feeling overexposed.'

Sheer: 'If you're going to wear sheer, invest in some great lingerie that's meant to be seen. Layering a sheer shirt over a funky bra is a decidedly confident, in-your-face look that is both feminine and modern.'

Sequins: 'Do yourself a favour. The next time you're in a store, try on a sequined dress and see how you feel. You'll stand a bit taller and you notice a slight sway to your walk.'

Satin: 'It's luxurious and sensual and it's got lots of flash. For a sophisticated and fitted look, try a stretch-satin vest and skirt.'

Red: 'The signature colour of divas everywhere, red ignites something in anyone who wears it. It's also a fabulous colour for accessories. A great pair of red shoes can add impact to any outfit.'

Gowns: 'If you want to have a ball, wear a gown. If it's versatility you want, try separates. Who said a gown has to be one-piece? Try a shantung silk or organza full skirt with a bustier or fitted camisole. Wearing a gown is like waving a magic wand over yourself. Pick the right one and something great is bound to happen.'

How Low Can You Go? A Word about Showing Breasts

Some celebrities' breasts attract so much attention they almost need an agent of their own. But to look stylish instead of porn-star tacky, the secret is to reveal just enough, but not too much.

Toupee tape is the tool-of-the-trade for keeping a star modest when the dress is far from it. When Jennifer Lopez wore that practically frontless green print Versace dress at the Grammys she relied on toupee tape (thicker than Sellotape and a lot stickier) that was stuck to both the fabric and her skin.

If your desire is to create more of a cleavage, then go for a bra that has padding on the outer edges of the cups to push the breasts together, or, if the top of the dress is too bare to wear a bra, invest in individual stick-on bra cups that can be strategically placed to offer that much-craved lift. Another solution is calling upon the services of a well-skilled tailor who can sew undergarments into evening-wear.

★ **STAR BOX** *Don't sleep on your front or side. It encourages the skin of the décolleté to crinkle and wrinkle. Lie flat and save your bust.*

---

20 SECRETS TO BECOMING A SAVVY SHOPPER

As we've learned, celebrities aren't necessarily born with great skin, hair or bodies. The same goes for great wardrobes. Although inbred style is pure instinct for some – Kate Hudson, Gwyneth Paltrow and Cameron Diaz readily spring to mind – leave others to style themselves and they can become a walking fashion disaster. Jennifer Aniston has learned this fast. In an interview with *Harper's Bazaar* she revealed, 'A couple of outfits I've worn were pointed out. One was just black pants paired with a black shirt. How do you screw that up? Somehow I did. Then I received some criticism for a dress I wore to the Emmys one year. It was beautiful, but slightly reminiscent of *Dynasty*. And once I was told that a jacket I'd worn looked like a lab coat, which it did. I had to get educated.'

Off the red carpet there's slightly less fashion pressure for celebrities, but with our insatiable hunger for pictures, they're now photographed putting out the rubbish, walking the dog and doing every other mundane duty you can think of. So looking well-dressed – or shabby but chic – 24/7 is an ongoing concern.

Luckily for celebrities, personal shoppers and stylists are there to serve them. If you don't have these invaluable people, what can you do? Here's some foolproof advice:

1. Pay attention to the pieces that you wear to death in your wardrobe and use them as inspiration. If that means wearing a pair of trousers that hug your butt perfectly, why not buy a pair in every colour?
2. Don't be dictated to by fashion. If it doesn't suit you, *don't buy it*.
3. Be true to your personality. Anything that's flashy, glitzy and attracts attention needs a big personality to carry off.
4. For soft and feminine pieces, try the lingerie department. Layering thin pretty vests can look great.
5. If you buy vintage (the modern word for second-hand), you can guarantee that someone will comment on it. It moves your look away from the expected and delivers distinction and style.
6. Unless you're mega thin, skip satin materials, as they can cling to lumps and bumps in all the wrong places. Stick to matt jersey.
7. Deep V-necks are the sexiest and most flattering necklines.
8. If your body isn't in the Zone, consider corsets, or 'shape-wear'. They shape the waist, pull in the stomach, smooth out the bottom and support the bust for a fabulous svelte silhouette.
9. Get your breasts measured. Many women buy a bra that's too small in the cup and too big around the back. It then offers no support, as the wrong parts are doing all the work.

10. Pick hipster jeans. They're far more flattering then high-waisted jeans. Wear them with a longer-length top if you're shy about showing off a midriff.

11. As with eyeshadow and lipstick, never let shoes fight for attention with a dress or vice versa. Match the shoes (at least the colour) to the outfit.

12. Unless you've got racehorse legs, avoid ankle straps. They shorten the look of the leg. And remember, celebrities never do tights, even if it's below freezing.

13. Avoid top-to-toe orange, white, green and pink, all of which can expand your shape. Colours that camouflage include neutrals, and colours that minimise and make you look slimmer are black, navy and grey.

14. Jiggly knees? Make sure your skirts hit below your knees, not on them. And if you're wearing long boots, ensure they don't end right below the knee, as this will draw attention to them.

15. If your neck isn't long and swanlike *à la* Gwyneth Paltrow, skip the chokers and opt for longer pendants. This draws the eye away from the neck and onto the cleavage. Elizabeth Hurley is never seen wearing a choker, but a pendant often dangles between her breasts!

16. Clutch bags always win over shoulder and handbags for evening glamour.

17. Sunglasses: the bigger, the darker, the better. The hidden eye undoubtedly says, 'I'm famous.' For star appeal wear them the entire time, even if it's snowing!

18. The same rule for jewellery. Don't be modest with your gems (fake or not). J-Lo doesn't sing about her 'rocks' for nothing.

19. Contrast belts with clothes. For instance wear a silver chain belt hung low on the waist over a jersey dress.

20. The ultimate accessory of them all? A good-looking man. All the better if he's famous in his own right. It spells double the exposure.

★ **STAR BOX** *Ever seen an A-lister with a thong showing? No. This look is for soap stars only. Keep your pants hidden and your mystery intact.*

Turn heads: how to ooze glamour

OK, you're leading the diva life: celebrity hairdresser, expensive sunglasses, luxury moisturiser and limos home (you're in the red, but hey, you'll be 'discovered' soon), but how do you go about being an out-and-out attention-grabber at a party or première? Bianca Jagger turned up on a horse at Studio 54 for her birthday bash in the seventies and Jennifer Lopez stole the scene at the Grammy Awards in 2000 when she wore a barely there Versace dress that left nothing to the imagination. However flashy the entrance or outrageous the outfit, you can't help admiring these divas.

> 'It is better to be looked over than overlooked.'
>
> **Mae West**

Although there is nothing more glamorous than controversy and whipping up a hullabaloo, the root of all glamour has to be confidence – and a generous dose of it. Everybody has the ability to light up an occasion, the question is how to use it. As the ultimate movie diva of them all says:

> 'I am not interested in money. I just want to be wonderful.'
>
> **Marilyn Monroe**

Here are a few confident and sexy tricks to get you started.

Don't Shy Away: There is a general feeling that people who cannot look you straight in the eye are untrustworthy or have something to hide. Whatever, minimal eye contact while conversing with someone is likely to project as a negative attitude. When you enter a room, walk in as though you deserve to be there, make a beeline for the friendliest face, hold their eye and smile. If you want to come across as flirtatious and sexual, look out from under your eyelashes.

Find Your Voice: Is your voice holding you back from stardom? Many a beautiful woman has been let down by her voice. Perhaps the most common vocal failing is to speak at a higher pitch than naturally fits the voice. Research shows speaking at the wrong pitch can keep you from drawing people in, but just a few words of greeting can raise the hairs on the neck if delivered in the right tones. Think of Kathleen Turner's bedroom voice. Soft and slow is the way to go. Speaking at a measured, controlled speed makes people listen. It shows you're calling the shots. A shrill, rushed and high-pitched voice can empty a room. Finally, if you want to make an impression, don't drone on and on. You'll make more impact if you say a few words and move on.

Ignore the Dress Code: Codes are there to be broken. Everybody wears the LBD. Be different. Be bold. Be photographed. But remember, never look scruffy!

Let Your Body Language Be Open: Whoever saw a diva being photographed with her arms folded as if she were chatting over the garden fence? People read this as a defensive, withdrawn position. Throw your arms wide to embrace your audience. Alternatively, throw out sensuality: stand with your hand resting on an exaggerated hip. This simple gesture shows off your figure to its full advantage.

Be Touchy Feely: Touch someone on the forearm when you say something. That person will remember it more than your perfume.

Be a Real Eye Opener: Half-shut eyes when out of the bedroom shout boredom. Make a beeline for someone that stimulates you. Your eyes will actually get wider and shine. Silently throw out strong sexual signals with a slow wink – if you're confident enough.

 STAR BOX *Retain an air of mystery. Interest is aroused by a diva who never apologises or explains.*

Girls on film: how to take a good picture

A picture has to be worth a thousand words. And that doesn't mean throwing your head back, braying like a donkey and kicking your legs up in the air. Celebrities have to learn to contain their emotions, even if they are happy to be taking home an Oscar. The bank of photographers at such events, armed and potentially dangerous with their supersonic lenses, have celebrities covered from every possible angle. A bad pose equals a bad and unflattering picture. Here are pointers that celebrities use to ensure they make lurve not war with the camera:

★ Smile straight at the camera. If you've got wrinkles, they'll look like laughter lines. If you're posing po-faced, they'll look like wrinkles!

★ If you're sitting down, avoid looking squat by lifting your head up to stretch your neck. Turn slightly away from the camera and look side on and up to the camera. This way everything falls back and into place.

★ Don't throw your head back and laugh if you have amalgam fillings.

★ This may look ridiculous off camera, but believe me it works. Stand with your hands on your hips and turn slightly to the side. Move your chest and neck forwards and stick your bottom out. This will stretch and angle your body something wonderful.

★ Don't look over your shoulder unless you want a necklace of a thousand crease lines under your jaw. The most flattering angle is to move your chin slightly down and to one side to define your bone structure. Your eyes should be glancing coyly off to the side.

★ If you're going sleeveless, place your arms about an inch (2.5cm) away from your body and slightly behind it to make them appear slimmer.

★ Avoid matronly-looking arms by not waving or hugging anyone. Arms will spread like jelly if not toned.

★ Avoid looking jowly by putting your tongue on the roof of your mouth.

★ Unless you aspire to be Pamela Anderson, add a slip underneath a chiffon dress or the flashbulbs will expose everything.

Spinning: coping with life's twists and turns

'Spin doctor': a modern term for skilful manipulation. Behind every great star there's a spin doctor ready to bully and flatter the media. So a celebrity has never been sacked, she's just decided to spend more quality time with her family. A celebrity never views herself as overweight, but as 'never happier' and 'more womanly' with 'curves in all the right places'. If her film is a box-office flop, that's because it's 'art'. You get the picture?

CELEBRITY PICKINGS *Winona's First-class Spin*
The very term 'spin' means to turnaround. And in this case for the better. Winona Ryder was caught on a shoplifting spree in Saks Fifth Avenue, but far from looking down and out in Beverly Hills, she turned up at court looking the picture of innocence: Alice band, high-buttoned coat and regal posture. Escaping a jail sentence, she was instead court-ordered to do community service, for which she received a glowing report, thereby endearing herself to everybody. Plus designer Marc Jacobs thought Winona looked so cute in his demure little

black-and-white dress at her trial that he decided to hire her
for his ad campaign. And they say crime doesn't pay!

The art to spinning with the best of them is learning how to elevate your life from ordinary to extraordinary. Catherine Zeta Jones is a prime example of this. A hard-working and ambitious dancer from the Mumbles in Wales, she has spun her life so well she's been rotating ever since. Quitting England after finishing *The Darling Buds of May*, she booked a one-way ticket to LA and, as they say, has never looked back. Networking relentlessly with hotshot directors, she landed roles in Hollywood block-busters such as *The Mask of Zorro* and *Entrapment* before meeting Hollywood royalty Michael Douglas. In just a few years she had spun herself from an unsophisticated jobbing actress to a woman with Hollywood at her feet. Likewise Madonna – after her ill-advised *Sex* book, when her popularity dipped, she spun herself enough to put her seedy past behind her and is now hailed as a devoted mother and wife who just happens to have a successful singing career too. Today she barely shows cleavage.

So what does it take to make people see your positive side? Our own personal success largely hinges on the attitudes we choose to adopt. Even the words we use to describe our situation can make a huge difference. Talking to yourself in positive or negative terms can go a long way towards shaping your future. It can pave the way for a more fulfilling and satisfying life. The same techniques that turn people into celebrities can help you face challenges too.

How to Psych Yourself Up for the Spotlight

★ Set goals. This is a serious business. Don't be fooled into thinking a celebrity just 'happened' to be handed her best part without working for it. Her goal-setting would have certainly been focused and turned into a game plan. You can do this too. When you say you're going to do something, do it. And tell people. That way you'll lose credibility with yourself and in the eyes of others if you don't. A little bit of outside pressure can even make you more determined to succeed. Go ahead and think big. Catherine Zeta Jones and Madonna did!

★ Don't view your goals as chores but choices. One way to do this is to stop believing that you're the only person who finds change unsettling. Change can be exciting, even if a little scary. Without change, nothing happens!

★ Move on from mistakes. What celebrity hasn't made wrong choices? Whether it's a dud film, the wrong dress or a boyfriend that made headlines for all the wrong reasons, they've learned you just have to move on from it and make better choices next time. Frustration, anger and disappointment can drain your energy, but keep imagining a 'stop' sign popping up into your head to remind yourself to let go of the past and look to the future. If you act as though you've forgotten about your mistake, others will too.

★ Listen to your critics. It can be hard to take criticism, but you can learn from it. No one likes to hear nega-tive feedback, whether it's a celebrity reading a less than rave review about her role in a film or you getting a sounding out from your boss. But they could be right. Hear your critics out before you decide whether to take their comments to heart.

★ Don't become envious about other people's success, become inspired. An envious person usually views themselves as incapable in some way, usually incapable of growth and change. The reality is, we're all capable of mastering new things. Gain new perspectives and you'll reach new heights.

★ You're without a man and see yourself as lonely. So what? Have Nicole Kidman, Minnie Driver and Renée Zellweger shied away from public life when single? Have they heck! No, they're looked upon by the public as wonderfully independent. Nicole may have had her dark days after splitting from Tom Cruise, but quickly spun herself to be a leading lady on her own merits.

★ We may think stars are too self-indulgent, but they see themselves as self-nurturing. If they're not going to look after themselves, who is? The same is true for you. Realise that taking care of yourself is an essential part of modern life. If you don't take the time to recharge, you'll eventually run out of energy. Feeling guilty about taking care of yourself can stem from lack of self-esteem. If that's the case, convince yourself you're worth it and book that day at the spa.

If All Else Fails, Adopt Your Own Celebrity Posse

Celebrities are always desperately seeking attention and no celebrity diva worth her diamonds relies on just herself.

When she jets in to promote a new film, she's hardly going to go unnoticed when rushed through the airport with around 20 hangers-on – or should I say 'entourage'? Nothing gets you noticed quicker than an entourage of people. And this tactic can be your last resort for attracting attention!

If there's one thing the stars know how to do, it's delegate, delegate, delegate. Initially, when just starting to seek out the spotlight, a star's 'team' usually consists of a few of their close friends, but as their fame levels increase so does the power of their posse. The diva has her well-tuned ear to the ground for helpers who will make her life bigger and better. The diva that is Jennifer Lopez has around 20 or more in her in crowd, including an eyebrow waxer. I've already covered the glamorisers – hairstylists, make-up artists and such like – but there's also the profound and sometimes disturbed celebrity soul to think about. Healers, head trippers and all-round handlers a go go all add the cachet of glamour to stars' lives and are seen as so crucial that many simply write the costs into their film contracts. Here's the checklist an A-lister regards as essential:

Personal Assistant. Also known as Dogsbody or All-round Doormat. They are shouted at, have mobiles thrown at their heads and are told they're useless. But they have the ability to mind-read what the star wants or needs. A PA is on call 24/7 and barely lasts more than a few seasons. Yes, they are as disposable as high fashion and there's always someone else more than ready to fill their shoes.

Agent. It's not surprising that some stars end up marrying their agents, as they are hard-headed, tough-talking go-getters and have nothing more taxing to think of than a star's welfare and bank balance – along with their own, of course.

Housekeeper. You don't think celebrities do their own housework or laundry, do you? They have a housekeeper and the housekeeper has cleaners working under her. Keeping a palatial home spotless is an expensive business.

Chef. As mentioned earlier, all super celebrities have to have a nutritionist. But once the diet is sorted, you don't expect them to cook it, do you? Jennifer Lopez apparently takes her chef everywhere, Madonna can't cook and won't cook so hires in one and Courteney Cox throws a dinner party twice a week and invites the chef – to cook!

Hot-shot Public Relations Guru. Hiring the best PR or publicist in showbiz is money well spent as far as getting the right coverage is concerned. These media manipulators announce break-ups and marriages and ensure that the stories the stars never want published are kept in the closet. When stars feel a little dowdy and sense they need to be seen in the right hangouts with the right person hanging off their arm, the PR person is the one they turn to to make them look hip. In essence, PRs are mean operators and manipulate the public in whichever way will benefit the celebrity.

Alternative Gurus. I could be talking palm-reading, colour therapy, Kabbala teachings, Apache Indian wisdom or just general spiritual fulfilment. The likes of Gwyneth Paltrow and Madonna have been known to seek psychic guidance on pressing topics like love, relationships and career moves. Surrounded by yes people, the famous can sometimes lose their sense of identity and seek these people out to find some meaning in their cocooned and very unreal lives. In fact stars can't get enough of New Age practices and therapies and are more than willing to pay for them. These gurus aren't millionaires for nothing! And in true Hollywood style it's said there's also an increase in demand for healing hairdressers and beauticians!

Acupuncturist, Masseuse, Chiropractor . . . The body beautiful has to be kept in fine working order and is forever lying under skilled and healing fingertips.

Bodyguards. The ultimate in showy accessories (real security is never conspicuous). A bling-bling bodyguard can also double up as a chauffeur or a beefy date if the star is in need of a 'prop'.

Nannies. Have you noticed the rich and famous only ever seem to employ plain-looking nannies? They don't want their husbands running off with them!

★ **STAR BOX** *Every diva thinks she is an original and has something to offer. Adopt this mindset too and see how different people react to you.*

---

quiz

ARE YOU READY TO LIVE THE CELEBRITY LIFE?

You've read the book, tried the tips, revamped your look and spun your life. But do you have the presence and attitude to wing it as your local celebrity? Take this fun test and find out:

1. When you order a meal in a restaurant do you:

a) Order a three-course meal and lick the plate?

b) Order off the menu and push half of it to the side of the plate?

c) Restaurant? You always order takeaways.

2. Which celebrity do you aspire to be like?

a) Any soap star – it must be great to open local supermarkets.

b) Sarah Jessica Parker – she looks fab both on and off screen.

c) Sandra Bullock – she doesn't take the celebrity life too seriously.

3. You're going to a party and are due for an appointment at the hairdresser's. Do you:

a) Skip the shampoo and just ask for a trim.

b) Request a sophisticated up-do you could never manage yourself at home.

c) Take your dress and shoes with you and ask for something subtle to complement them.

4. Your underwear drawer consists of:

a) Pants that would shame you if you were run over by a bus.

b) Expensive lingerie – and this is a luxury you have no intention of dropping (except for the right man!)

c) It's a mix of big pants and small – depends how lucky you feel!

5. Admit it – have you ever dragged your favourite outfit out of the laundry basket?

a) All the time.

b) Never.

c) Sometimes.

6. Which three words describe you?

a) Dependable, secure, sheltered.

b) Dynamic, hedonistic, feminine.

c) Natural, loving, happy.

7. What's your happy-hour thirst quencher?

a) Half a pint of larger.

b) Vodka martini.

c) Chilled Chardonnay.

8. Which night would rock for you?

a) A night in eating crisps on the sofa with a video.

b) Cocktails, swish eateries, an attention-seeking crowd.

c) A spontaneous night out. It's the positive energy that makes you happy, whether it's a hip party or dinner for two.

9. What's your fitness routine?
a) Walking the dog.
b) A personal trainer called Carlos.
c) The local gym.

10. Where do you shop?
a) The Internet. It's so convenient.
b) All the big-name stores mixed with a little vintage.
c) The shopping mall.

YOUR SCORE:

Mostly As
You admire celebrity from a distance, devour the gossip but can't ever imagine entering that distant world of glamour and glitz – although you secretly yearn to copy their style now and again. Add glamour to your life by booking in for a new hairdo, revamping your make-up and poring over fashion magazines for style inspiration. Stop looking upon your life as a routine and start living it – glamorously.

Mostly Bs
You don't just live a celebrity life, you play a leading role in it. Indulgent and dynamic, you're a woman whose vibrant energy is infectious. A highly polished look is part of who you are and you love nothing more than taking centre stage. Loaded with enthusiasm and sometimes larger than life, you burn with desire and are often the life and soul of the party. Is your name Madonna, by any chance?

Mostly Cs

You class yourself as a Sandra Bullock (in fact you opted for her in question two). Celebrity entices you, but you're never happier than in your own environment. You smile from the inside out and tend to lean towards the simple pleasures in life. You don't actively seek to get noticed, but as plenty of TLC, the newest fragrance and a great hair colour are always right at the top of your beauty wish list, you can't help but turn heads. But keeping abreast of the new trends is more important to you than being photographed in them.

Resources

UK HOT SPOTS

Hair Salons
Daniel Hersheson
45 Conduit Street
London W1R 9FB
Tel: 020 7434 1747

Richard Ward
162b Sloane Street
London SW1X 9BS
Tel: 020 7245 6151

Colourist
Jo Hansford
19 Mount Street
London W1Y 5RA
Tel: 020 7495 7774

Teeth Whitening

Capital Dental
298 Fulham Road
Chelsea
London SW10 9EP
Tel: 0800 587 7962

Facialist

Leonard Drake Skin Care Centres
8 Lancer Square
Kensington Church Street
London W8 4EH
Tel: 020 7937 7060
and
The Cloisters Mail
Kingston upon Thames
Surrey KT1 1RS
Tel: 020 8541 0999

Personal Training

Absolute Fitness
Tel: 020 7834 0000

Body Control Pilates
6 Langley Street
London WC2H 9JA
Tel: 020 7379 3734
www.bodycontrol.co.uk

Alternative
The Joshi Clinic
57 Wimpole Street
London W1G 8YP
Tel: 020 7487 5456

Cosmetic Surgeon
Laurence Kirwan
112 Harley Street
London W1G 7JQ
Tel: 020 7908 3860

AUSTRALIAN HOT SPOTS

Spas
Jurlique Wellness Sanctuary Day Spa
Como Centre
nr Chapel Street & Toorak Road
South Yarra 3141
Melbourne
Tel: 63 (0) 9827 0755

Spa Chakra
6 Cowper Wharf Road
Woolloomooloo
New South Wales NSW 2011
Tel: + 02 9368 0888
www.chakra.net.spa

Hair Salon
Valonz Haircutters
10 William Street
Paddington
Sydney
Tel: (02) 9360 2444

Beauty Junkie Store
Miss Frou Frou
20–22 Elizabeth Street
Paddington
Sydney
Tel: (02) 9360 2869

Hair Removal
The Australian Laser Clinic
www.laserclinic.com.au

NEW ZEALAND HOT SPOTS

Day Spa
L'unova
48 Broadway
Newmarket
Auckland
Tel: (09) 520 6731

Hairdresser
Glint
159 Hurstmere Road

Takapuna
North Shore
Auckland
Tel: (09) 489 9058

Best for Botox
Dr Catherine Stone
The Face Place
Level 2
10 Vulcan Lane
Auckland
Tel: 0800 2BOTOX

Best Store for Beauty Junkies
Glamourpuss
290a Broadway
Newmarket
Auckland
Tel: (09) 524 4741

SOUTH AFRICAN HOT SPOTS

Health and Beauty Clinic
Aromabar
23 Derry Street
Vredehoek
Cape Town 8001
Tel: (021) 461 6610

Spa
S.K.I.N. Wellness Spa
Dock Road
V&A Waterfront
Cape Town 8001
Tel: (021) 425 3551
www.skinonline.co.za

Hair Salon
Isjon Intercoiffure
Tel: (011) 805 4655

Cosmetic Surgeon
Dr Des Fernandes
822 Fountain Medical Centre
Heerengracht Centre
Cape Town 8001
Tel: (021) 425 2310

RECOMMENDED READING

Phillip Bloch, *Elements of Style*, Little, Brown, 1998
Dr Nicholas Perricone, *The Perricone Prescription*, Thorsons, 2003
Simon Waterson, *Commando Workout*, Thorsons, 2002

RECOMMENDED WEBSITES

www.gunnarpeterson.com for secrets of celebrity workouts
www.bodydoctorfitness.com for celebrity workouts
www.etonline.com/celebrity for the best celebrity gossip and interviews

Index